The Diploma in Child Health

A practical study guide
Volume 2

By Dr Anil Garg, Dr Siba Prosad Paul,
Dr Geethika Bandaranayake, Dr Urmilla Pillai,
Dr Neelu Garg and Daniel Barry

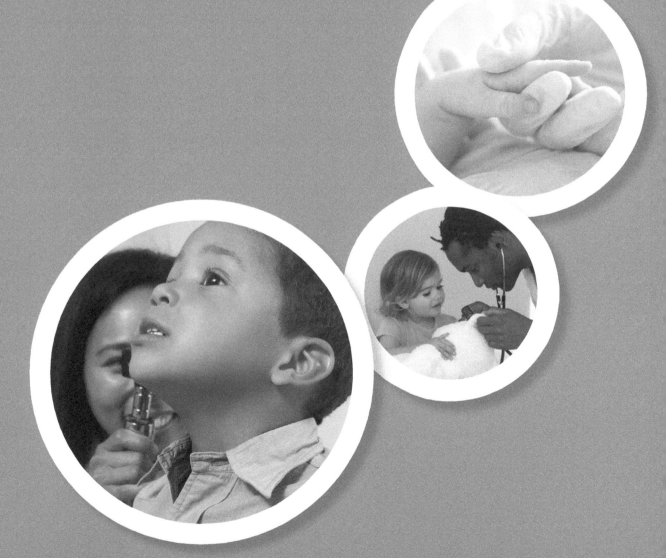

Diploma in Child Health: A practical study guide, volume 2

Published by:
Pavilion Publishing and Media Ltd
Rayford House
School Road
Hove
East Sussex
BN3 5HX
Tel: 01273 434 943
Fax: 01273 227 308
Email: info@pavpub.com

Published 2014

A catalogue record for this book is available from the British Library.

Print ISBN: 978-1-909810-78-5
Epub ISBN: 978-1-909810-79-2
PDFebook ISBN: 978-1-909810-80-8
Kindle ISBN: 978-1-909810-81-5

Pavilion is the leading training and development provider and publisher in the health, social care and allied fields, providing a range of innovative training solutions underpinned by sound research and professional values. We aim to put our customers first, through excellent customer service and value.

Authors: Anil Garg, Siba Paul, Geethika Bandaranayake, Urmilla Pillai, Neelu Garg and Daniel Barry
Production editor: Mike Benge, Pavilion Publishing and Media Ltd
Cover design: Phil Morash, Pavilion Publishing and Media Ltd
Page layout and typesetting: Phil Morash, Pavilion Publishing and Media Ltd
Printing: Ashford Colour Press Ltd., Gosport, Hants.

Contents

Preface

The DCH examination consists of both written and clinical components, and this book and its counterpart, Volume 1, are intended to help candidates prepare for the clinical examination and guide you through the various stations you will encounter.

I would suggest that you use the guides to practise under examination conditions and not use them as bedtime reading. The cases are real and cover a wide cross-section of potential topics. It is important to note that the books are not intended to be textbooks, and although they supply some basic information on the topics covered, you will need to do some extensive supportive reading.

This is Volume 2, which covers the data interpretation station, safe prescribing and structured oral stations. Volume 1 covers the remaining stations, which are common to both the DCH and the MRCPCH examinations.

I hope you find the books helpful to your preparations for the examination, and stimulating and informative reads.

I would like to take this opportunity to thank all of my colleagues who have contributed to these books and acknowledge the hard work they have put in to make them possible.

Remember, there is always room for improvement – practise, practise, practise…

Dr Anil Garg

Foreword

It is a pleasure to write a foreword to this book, which I'm sure will be warmly welcomed by junior doctors preparing for the DCH clinical examination. This examination is important for doctors wanting to demonstrate competency in looking after children in primary care settings, and for that reason is a valuable qualification to obtain.

The most recent format of the examination came into force in 2011, introducing new stations including safe prescribing, data interpretation and structured oral stations. The examination circuit is completed by having assessments of clinical skills, neurodisability and development and communication.

I found it interesting that the authors have decided to publish this book in two volumes, separating out the stations unique to the DCH clinical examination in one volume and having the stations common to that and the MRCPCH clinical examination in the other.

Together, these books provide a valuable resource for anyone preparing for the DCH examination, and Volume 1 will be a helpful tool for those taking the MRCPCH exam, as each station is considered separately and many clinical scenarios are presented within each section.

Anna Mathew
Consultant Paediatrician
Western Sussex hospitals NHS Trust, UK

Introduction:
The DCH examination

Children are a vulnerable group in society. They differ from adults in a number of ways, starting out as helpless and totally dependent on their carers for survival, and they have different needs due to the demands of growth and development. Although, comparatively, they make up a smaller proportion of the population than adults, they require much higher levels of care. Their needs are often quite specific and the people caring for them need special skills to provide for them.

The Diploma in Child Health (DCH) is a qualification that recognises that the holder has achieved the competencies and skills required to look after children. The examination has evolved over the years, both in format and in relevance. In the UK, it used to be the only qualification in paediatrics for hospital specialists taken after getting the Membership of the College of Physicians (MRCP). However, with the inception by Royal Charter in 1996 of the RCPCH (Royal College of Paediatrics and Child Health), membership of RCPCH (ie. the MRCPCH exams) established a second specialist qualification in addition to the DCH that confirms and attests a speciality in paediatrics.

The DCH used to be an examination run by hospital paediatricians for hospital paediatricians. In the UK, however, it has evolved into an examination oriented towards primary care and general practice. According to the RCPCH, the DCH is now designed to recognise competence in the care of children in general practitioner vocational trainees, staff grade doctors and senior house officers in paediatrics, as well as trainees in specialties allied to paediatrics.

The examination has a syllabus that encompasses paediatric care both in and out of hospital, plus services available and used outside the hospital settings. Examiners include hospital paediatricians, community paediatricians, general practitioners, paediatric surgeons and child psychiatrists.

This change in emphasis is important. In terms of the workload in primary care for a GP, children contribute approximately 30%, significantly more than their number in the community. GPs need to work with numerous agencies now involved in the multidisciplinary approach to childcare, and they need to recognise when to seek assistance from the appropriate agencies.

A busy GP has to manage children with acute and chronic conditions, monitor their development, discuss health promotion and be aware of child protection issues and various other screening programs. They also have to be aware of the resources available and how to tap them for the benefit of children they are looking after. Competence and confidence in dealing with them and their conditions are therefore vital.

The Diploma in Child Health is an accepted specialist qualification overseas. Hence it is important to have adequate experience of hospital paediatrics to pass the examination in the various domains: clinical, communication, history and management, development, prescribing and structured oral.

The safe prescribing station is a new domain in the exam, and has been introduced to improve prescribing skills and prevent harm to patients. Prescribing errors are in fact a leading cause of death in young adults between 18–45 years, after accidents. And it is not only prescribing errors, but errors in dispensing due to illegibility that also contribute to the total damage, hence the need for improvement. When prescribing, it is important to use the British National Formulary for Children (BNFC) to check for appropriate drug choice, dosage, side effects and interactions. There may be local guidelines available that can be used instead.

Candidates taking the DCH examination overseas must be aware of the management and support provided to children in the community in which they practise. They should read up on and be aware of the management and support that is available in the UK. This will often not be available overseas, but it can be quoted as best practice and what should be aspired to in the future, and contrasted with what is actually available.

The structure of the exam

The DCH examination consists of two parts:

Foundation of Practice: Part 1. This is the written component and is the same as that for MRCPCH. There are two papers consisting of multiple choice, extended matching and best-of-five format questions. The written questions are prepared and checked in different settings before being used in the examination. After each diet, the performance of each question is evaluated and each question is given a score. Poorly discriminating questions are not used in the future.

Clinical examination: Part 2. This is the practical component of the examination and has been included since 2006. It has evolved from a format that included a long case, short cases and viva, to an OSCE (Objective Structured Clinical Examination) format, which is more consistent in assessment, fairer to candidates and has improved accountability. A number of candidates are assessed in the same 'station/skill set' by the same examiner with the same patient, to provide better consistency in assessment and grading.

The RCPCH puts a great deal of effort into ensuring that every examination is of a comparable standard to the last and is thorough and fair. Setting standards is an important part of ensuring fairness and equality across the various centres hosting the examination. It involves deciding on what is expected of the candidate with reference to the anchor statements as published by the RCPCH. The communication and prescribing scenarios are 'standard set' at the RCPCH, and guidance is given to the centres hosting the examination, thus reducing variability in assessment.

Before an exam, the examiners are given a written summary of the signs and symptoms of the clinical cases that are to be investigated during the examination. Children are then assessed at the examination centre for the validity of these symptoms and a standard is set by two examiners, who determine what is expected of a candidate in order to achieve a particular grade from 'clear pass' to 'clear fail'. 'Unacceptable' is reserved for rare cases. These standard setting forms are returned to the RCPCH at the end of the examination.

The stations

In the DCH clinical examination, skills and competence are assessed in seven different areas at eight stations. These cover:

- communication
- focused history and management
- structured oral
- clinical assessment
- child development
- data interpretation
- safe prescribing.

The eight OSCE stations are divided into two circuits – separated as follows:

Circuit A (lasts 36 minutes): each station lasts six minutes with a three-minute interval between stations.

Circuit B (lasts 48 minutes): each station lasts nine minutes with a three-minute interval between stations.

The candidates move from station to station while the examiner remains at the same station during the session. This provides consistency in examining and marking the performance of the candidates against the standard that was set before the start of the session.

There is a 40 minute break between the two circuits.

12 objective assessments are made of each candidate. One assessment is made at each station in Circuit A (for a total of four assessments), and two assessments are made at each station in Circuit B (for a total of eight assessments).

Circuit A grid

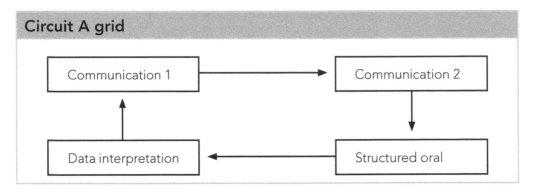

| Communication 1 | → | Communication 2 |
| Data interpretation | ← | Structured oral |

Time frame for Circuit A

Station	Interval outside	In station	Warning
Communication 1	Scenario available Read and make plan	6 minute assessment	1 minute remaining
Communication 2	Scenario available Read and make plan	6 minute assessment	1 minute remaining
Data interpretation	No information available outside	2 minutes to interpret data 4 minute discussion with examiner	1 minute remaining
Structured oral	No information available outside	1–2 minutes to read scenario 4–5 minutes discussion with examiner	1 minute remaining

For more information, visit www.rcph.ac.uk/examinations/dch

Circuit B grid

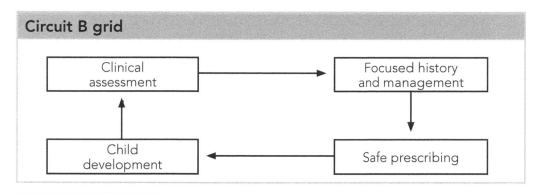

Time frame for Circuit B

Station	Interval outside	In station	Warning
Clinical assessment	None	Assessment of child 6 min Discussion with examiner 3 min	1 minute remaining
Focused history/ management	Scenario to read *Read and make plan*	6 min with role player Role player leaves 3 min discuss with examiner	4 minutes remaining
Development	None	6 min assess child 3 min discuss with examiner	4 minutes remaining
Prescribing	Task description *Read and make plan*	5 minute to write prescription 4 min discussion with examiner	5 minutes remaining

Note – Two sets of marks are awarded for each station (for task and discussion)

Marking schedule

Grade	Marks	Description
Clear pass (CP)	12	Satisfied requirements and excelled
Pass	10	Some minor failings – not as good as expected
Bare fail	8	Inappropriate number of minor or some important errors
Clear fail	4	Poor performance
Unacceptable	0	Unprofessional behaviour – rough, rude

Total of 120 marks are needed in examination to be awarded a pass.

Clinical examination station

The following are some examples of tasks that you might be asked to perform at the clinical examination station:

A: 'Please examine Peter's chest. He is eight years old and has come for review due to his recurrent cough.'

B: 'Please examine Anu, five years old, who had a murmur noted during a febrile illness four weeks ago.'

C: 'Joanna is seven years old and her mother is worried about her walking, believing she has a limp. Please examine Joanna's legs.'

D: 'Daniel, six years old, has come for review as his mother feels he is not as good with his hands as his twin sister. Can you please do a fine motor assessment?'

The examiner will complete the mark sheet as the candidate proceeds with the task at the station, and will write comments about the performance for later feedback and in case there are any questions as to why a certain mark was given.

Data interpretation station

Data interpretation is a new station in the DCH, which tests the ability of a candidate to assess the results of investigations in a clinical setting. The data interpretation station has one scenario only, which will consist of a set of results from a haematology or biochemistry report, for example, or from an audiogram or a renogram etc. The candidate's task is to interpret the data provided, work out a differential diagnosis if appropriate, devise a management plan and discuss it with the examiner.

It is rare for identical questions to appear but there are recurring themes.

Marks are awarded against a pre-determined standard, and will assess whether a candidate:

- identifies the problem
- accurately interprets the data in the clinical context provided
- achieves the correct diagnosis or a differential diagnosis
- is fluent and confident in discussing management of the condition
- demonstrates their knowledge underpinning good paediatric practice
- demonstrates a good understanding of the evidence base ie. NICE guidelines.

There is no substitute for a broad knowledge base and an ability to think laterally. Remember, the data could be normal or could indicate significant pathology.

Safe prescribing station

Safe prescribing is a station for assessing the understanding of pharmacological agents, other compounds, devices and measures used in managing disease conditions, both acute and chronic. A clinical scenario is given and the candidate has to prescribe the most appropriate drug or device. Competences assessed include the correct use of medication/intervention in the right medical context and in the correct dosage. The candidate has to decide on the most appropriate strategy and write out a prescription with the help of the BNFC (British National Formulary for Children) (if overseas, local guidelines may be used). This is followed by a discussion with the examiner.

Latest updates can be obtained from the RCPCH – http://www.rcpch.ac.uk/Examinations/DCH

The structure of this study manual

In the subsequent sections of this study manual we will cover the following stations:

■ Safe prescribing

■ Data interpretation

■ Structured oral

In *The Diploma in Child Health: A practical study guide, volume 1*, the remaining stations are covered. These are:

■ Communication

■ Clinical assessment

■ Focused history and management

■ Child development

The books have been divided in this way because the stations covered in this manual are only relevant to the DCH exam. The stations covered by volume 1 are relevant to both the DCH and the MRCPCH exam and is therefore relevant to candidates taking either.

The difference between the DCH and MRCPCH examinations lies in the degree of competence expected, which is reflected in the time allocated for testing competencies at each station.

The scenario-based approach that is used in this manual keeps in perspective that the candidate is a new GP in the UK who has four to six months' of working in paediatrics and other specialities during their two years' hospital-based training and one year in general practice. During this time, the individual will have acquired other common and transferrable competences from the various other specialities they have developed through their vocational training.

The scenarios in this manual are generally designed to be practised with another person who can act as a 'role player', either playing the part of the patient or their parent, or the examiner in scenarios where you will have to discuss your findings. The information for each scenario is therefore divided into different sections, some of which both you and your partner will have access to, and the rest which will only be available to the role player.

In scenarios where the role player is playing the examiner, they will essentially have the 'answers', and a list of areas that the examiner will be looking for.

The scenarios are presented in four sections, each in a different coloured box:

- The first box sets the scene and outlines the task you need to perform as the candidate.

- The information in the second box will vary depending on the station. It will contain either:
  - the information given to the role player, which should not be available to the candidate
  - further, more detailed information for the candidate, such as a set of data to be interpreted or the details of a clinical examination.

- The third box, which should not be available to the candidate, contains information about what the examiner expects of a candidate and, usually, the 'answers' or conclusions that the candidate would be expected to reach.

- The fourth box contains some further basic information on the topic that may be useful for other stations, or that might simply further the candidates' understanding of the topic.

- Finally, there is a small space for you to make notes that come to mind.

We therefore recommend that you do not use the book as a passive reading material, but work through it with friends in small study groups using the book as a guide.

However, if you do not have a study partner you can still work through the scenarios by simply covering up or ignoring those boxes that contain information for the role player, and writing down your responses, diagnoses and thoughts. These can then be checked against the information or answers in the remaining boxes.

Further video resources to help you can be found at www.mrcpchclinicals.org

General approach to the examination

By their very nature, examinations are very artificial situations, far removed from the day-to-day routines we all are so accustomed to. On a normal day, one would come to work and get on with the tasks as they arise: handover, ward round, admitting, taking a history from a parent or patient and working out a management plan, multidisciplinary meeting, talking to children or parents, and if there is more than one job to be done, we prioritise. Sometimes we might demonstrate our skills to our junior colleagues for them to learn, or to seniors to get their feedback with a view to improving and providing better care to our patients, but generally we are not concerned about who is watching us and we do not have to show our best side.

Examinations, however, are different. Think of the driving test you may have taken. It was not only about your driving; you had to 'exaggerate' your actions – adjusting the rear view mirror before starting, constantly checking mirrors and making sure it was noted by the examiner. It was not simply what you were doing that mattered, but also about *showing*, and ensuring that what you had been doing was noted.

Clinical examinations in general, and the DCH in particular, are not miles away from this. You have to 'perform', and to show off your various skills and competences in the different settings of the examination stations, be it communication with parents or a child or both, discussing with a colleague, taking a focused history, interpreting a result, or writing a prescription.

I, like most people, feel uncomfortable when I am being observed critically while doing something. It makes me nervous and jittery. In a work environment I can request an observer – such as a parent whose child is undergoing a lumbar puncture or a venepuncture – to kindly leave and wait outside while I complete the task. One does not have that option during an examination. Being observed is part of the deal we have agreed to, and coping with the nerves is an important factor in the final outcome.

Your preparation for the DCH examination will culminate at the examination centre, but should start much earlier: check out the route to the centre the night before, get a good night's sleep, leave yourself plenty of time to get ready, dress in a conservative style and present a professional image. Stay calm on the way to the examination centre and get there in good time as any delay or potential delays will increase your tension and anxiety, adversely affecting your ability to perform at your best.

As discussed, there are eight stations to negotiate including two communication stations during the examination and it is very unlikely that all of them will go completely to your satisfaction. There will be times when you think you have 'bombed' a particular station and the feeling is devastating. But it is very important not to lose your cool and go to pieces. My boss used to say, take it like a game of cricket – each station is one wicket – just because one or even two wickets fall with not enough score on the board, it does not mean the game is lost. Keep your head down, keep your concentration and try and score in the next station/wicket. The previous station cannot affect the next if you do not let it, and marks from one station can compensate for the other stations and take you to the desired total to pass. You should therefore never give up!

Communication is key to this examination. It is important in all sections and stations. You will be replying to questions throughout the examination. It is important to have a strategy that will guide you through most situations and keep you in control.

'That is a very good question!' is probably not the best response to come out with in the examination, though you may hear it time and again in the media.

Here are some essential tips.

- Do not be tempted to speak immediately after the question has been asked.

- Do not say the first thing that comes to mind – other ideas may not follow.

- Take up to 10 seconds to think over a question carefully.

- Work out precisely what is being asked.

- Differentiate from what you think you would like to have heard.

- Think of three common points in relation to the question asked.

- If possible, think of the next question that may follow on from your answer.

- Try to guide the examiner to areas you know well.

- If it so happens that you do not know enough about a particular condition, do not mention it – as long as it is not the first on the list.

- If you do not know something, admit your lack of knowledge and the examiner will move on – do not bluff – examiners are seasoned players.

- When you do start replying, keep your thoughts five seconds ahead of your mouth. With practice this is possible, difficult as it may seem now. Practising the scenarios in this manual with friends/study partners will get you used to this.

- Finally, if you are not sure of what is being asked – CLARIFY.

You may think that an initial five to 10-second silence is long, awkward and feels like eternity, but trust me, a 10-second silence in the middle of a sentence, when the ideas you want to convey are at the tip of your tongue but just won't come, is a lot more awkward and 'deafening'. You can try it with a recording.

This emphasis on communication is not 'overkill', and the time you spend now on practising and improving this skill will help you more than anything else you may do so close to the exam.

Remember, practice makes perfect – failing to prepare is preparing to fail.

We hope you find the book useful and interesting.

Data interpretation station

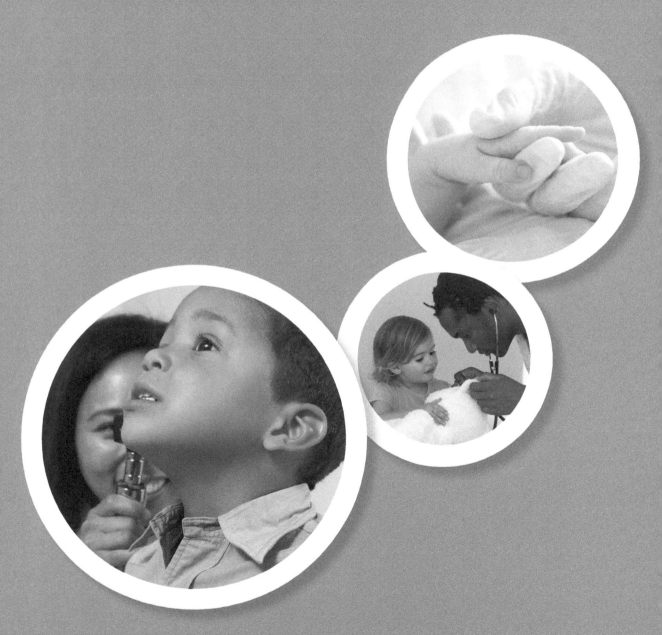

Data interpretation station

In the practice of modern medicine, our clinical interpretations are supported by data from a variety of laboratory results, be they haemotology, radiology or electrophysiology, for example. Using this information, we make decisions for the safe and effective management of the patients we care for. Logical and accurate interpretations of the data these tests supply are therefore important, both for clinical care and for success in the DCH examination.

At the data interpretation station you will be provided with a brief clinical scenario and then given results of an investigation related to a clinical problem. Your task is to digest this information in the context of the case history and reach a diagnosis and brief management plan. You will then have to discuss your conclusions with the examiner.

In this section, the second box supplies you with the data to be interpreted and then sets out a number of questions. The answers to these questions are in the third box and if working with a study partner they should be the only person with access to them.

If working alone, record your own interpretation before checking it against the answers.

Data interpretation station: case 1

Anaemia

Information given to the candidate

Abdul, five years old, has come back for review for his constipation. He passes blood with his stools at times.

Your task

Please see the data provided below.

You have two minutes to analyse the data and then four minutes to discuss your interpretation and management, if appropriate, with the examiner.

Data provided

Hb	9.5 g/dL – 95g/L
WBC	$7.8 \times 10^9/L$
Plats	$401 \times 10^9/L$
RBC	$4.8 \times 10^{12}/L$
Hct	31%
MCV	64 fL
MCH	19.6 pg
MCHC	30.5 g/dL
RDW	14%
Neut	$3.7 \times 10^9/L$
Lymph	$3.3 \times 10^9/L$
Mono	$0.4 \times 10^9/L$
Eosn	$4:0 \times 10^9/L$
Baso	$0.1 \times 10^9/L$

Questions

What are the abnormalities and what is your working diagnosis?

What would you do?

What advice will you give Abdul's parents?

What is expected from the candidate

The candidate should:

- identify any abnormalities in the results
- think of a differential diagnosis
- identify that it is most likely to be diet related
- establish safety net to recheck investigations for other conditions.

Answers

What are the abnormalities and what is your working diagnosis?

- Low haemoglobin, low haematocrit.
- Low MCV, low MCHC.
- Microcytic, hypochromic anaemia.

What would you do?

- Investigate diet, blood loss and constipation.
- Treat constipation, give iron supplements.
- Review in four weeks – recheck FBC, coeliac screen, ESR, CRP.
- It is important to rule out coeliac disease and possible inflammatory bowel disease.

What advice will you give Abdul's parents?

- Give medicine regularly.
- Decrease milk in diet and encourage solid foods.
- It is important to bring Abdul back for repeat blood tests in four weeks.

Further information

Iron deficiency can be caused by:

- an iron-poor diet – the most common cause
- poor iron absorption – coeliac disease
- long-term, slow blood loss – bleeding in the digestive tract.

Cow's milk consumption is a common cause of iron deficiency. It contains less iron than many other foods and also reduces iron absorption from other foods.

Iron is important, not only for haemoglobin production but also for general well-being, healthy hair and skin, and long-term development.

For more information, see:

http://www.nlm.nih.gov/medlineplus/ency/article/007134.htm

http://www.nhs.uk/conditions/Anaemia-iron-deficiency-/Pages/Introduction.aspx

For your notes and thoughts

Data interpretation station: case 2

Blood gas – respiratory acidosis in bronchiolitis

Information given to the candidate

Asim is an eight-week-old baby. He was born prematurely at 32^{+3} weeks and stayed in the local neonatal unit for five weeks. He needed CPAP support for the initial 48 hours and remained on oxygen for the first week of life.

He has currently been admitted with a clinical diagnosis of bronchiolitis and needs nasal cannula oxygen and is fed with a nasogastric tube. As his oxygen requirement is gradually increasing (FiO_2 0.55%) and he was noted to be head bobbing, a capillary blood gas test was carried out by the nurse looking after him.

Your task

Please see the data provided below.

You have two minutes to analyse the data and then four minutes to discuss your interpretation and management, if appropriate, with the examiner.

Data provided

Blood gas

pH	7.16
pCO_2	9.2 kPa
pO_2	3.5 kPa
BE	(+)7.5 mmol/L
HCO_3	32.2 mmol/L

Questions

What are the abnormalities and what is your working diagnosis?

What would you do?

What advice will you give Asim's parents?

What is expected from the candidate

The candidate should:
- identify abnormalities in the data
- have a differential diagnosis
- discuss management in a logical sequence.

Answers

What are the abnormalities and what is your working diagnosis?
- Low pH, high pCO_2, raised bicarbonate.
- Respiratory acidosis.
- Respiratory acidosis with metabolic compensation in an infant with bronchiolitis.

What would you do?
- Discuss with a senior colleague (eg. a registrar) and initiate either high flow oxygen therapy (via vapotherm/optiflow device) or start nasal CPAP.
- Monitor blood gas every four to six hours to review progress.
- Assess hydration status and if tolerated continue NGT feeds at 100mls/kg/day every two hours.
- If the infant is deteriorating, intravenous fluids may be needed (ideally 0.9% NaCl + 5% dextrose or 0.45% NaCl + 5% dextrose).
- Other management strategies in similar cases include a chest x-ray and intravenous antibiotics.
- Nasopharyngeal aspirate to detect the respiratory virus (high incidence of **respiratory syncitial virus** in this age group). RSV –ve bronchiolitis is also common. It is important for public health epidemiology and there is some association with asthma in older children.

What advice will you give Asim's parents?
- Explain the clinical condition.
- Reassure Asim's parents that he will get better but will need symptomatic support.

For your notes and thoughts

Data interpretation station: case 3

Cow's milk protein allergy

Information given to the candidate

Ruby, four months old, is seen for poor weight gain. She weighs 4kg and she takes five feeds per day, approximately 120–150ml per feed, of cow's milk based formula. She has not been weaned. She and her older brother have eczema. On examination she is well apart from this.

Your task

Please see the data provided below.

You have two minutes to analyse the data and then four minutes to discuss your interpretation and management, if appropriate, with the examiner.

Data provided

Haemoglobin	90.0 g/L – 9.0 g/dl
Platelets	320 x 10⁹/L
WBC	8.1 x 10⁹/L
Neutrophils	4.5 x 10⁹/L (2.0 – 7.5)
Lymphocytes	2.0 x 10⁹/L (1.5 – 4.0)
Monocytes	0.48 x 10⁹/L (0.3 – 0.8)
Eosinophils	1.5 x 10⁹/L (0.04 – 0.4)
Basophils	0.02 x 10⁹/L (0.01 – 0.1)
Anti-tissue transglutaminase Ab	-ve
Anti-endomyseal Ab	-ve
Jejunal biopsy	Villous atrophy

Questions

What are the abnormalities and what is your working diagnosis?

What would you do?

What advice will you give Ruby's parents?

What is expected from the candidate

The candidate should:

- identify the abnormalities
- not jump to diagnosis of coeliac disease as biopsy showed villous atrophy
- discuss results logically.

Answers

What are the abnormalities and what is your working diagnosis?

- Low haemoglobin – however, probably normal for her age.
- High eosinophil count.
- Vilious atrophy.
- Cow's milk protein intolerance.
- Failure to thrive.
- Malabsorption due to small bowel disease.

What would you do?

- Arrange to see dietitian.
- Start on extensively hydrolysed formula milk or amino-acid based formula.
- Give emollients for skin.

What advice will you give Ruby's parents?

- Discuss cow's milk protein allergy.
- Recommend the use of special milk formula.
- Review Ruby in two weeks.

Further information

The common symptoms of CMPA are:

- vomiting/reflux
- diarrhoea/constipation
- poor weight gain
- eczema.

In cases of CMPA there is often a family history of atopy.

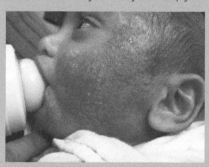

Raised eosinophil count and serum IgE levels are non-specific associated abnormalities.

Villious atrophy on jejunal biopsy is not diagnostic of coeliac disease and can also be caused by:

- soya protein intolerance
- gastroenteritis
- transient gluten intolerance
- giardiasis
- severe combine immune deficiency
- cytotoxic chemotherapy.

For more information, see: http://www.ncbi.nlm.nih.gov/pmc/articles/PMC1544422/

For your notes and thoughts

Data interpretation station: case 4

Coeliac disease

Information given to the candidate

Anna is a 13-year-old girl who has come for a follow-up. She was diagnosed with coeliac disease at the age of three years.

Your task

Please see the data provided below.

You have two minutes to analyse the data and then four minutes to discuss your interpretation and management, if appropriate, with the examiner.

Data provided

Haemoglobin	127 g/L – 12.7 g/dl
WCC	5.1 x 10^9/L
Platelets	242 x 10^9/L
TSH	2.88 (0.7–6.4mIu/L)
Coeliac screen	- ve
Weight	41.1 kg (25th–50th centile)
Height	159.9 cm (25th–50th centile)

Questions

What are the abnormalities and what is your working diagnosis?

What would you do?

What advice will you give Anna and her parents?

What is expected from the candidate

The candidate should:

- demonstrate a good understanding of coeliac disease – its presentation and diagnosis
- highlight good management – the need for multidisciplinary support, including input from a dietitian
- understand that a biopsy is the gold standard for diagnosis but that tTg is a good screening test
- explain that it will be necessary to follow-up throughout life
- advise regular monitoring for other autoimmune conditions such as diabetes mellitus or hypothyroidism.

Answers

What are the abnormalities and what is your working diagnosis?

- Normal haemoglobin.
- Normal thyroid screen.
- Normal coeliac screen.

What would you do?

- Refer to a dietitian and discuss a gluten-free diet.
- Explain good compliance with this diet.
- Reassure her and arrange to see in one year's time.

What advice will you give Anna and her parents?

- Provide reassurance.
- Emphasise importance of following a gluten-free diet.
- Explain/discuss the importance of a thyroid screen due to autoimmune nature of coeliac disease and hence checking for other possible comorbidities.

Further information

Coeliac disease is an autoimmune condition causing malabsorption. A combination of a person's genetic make-up and environment appear to play a part. It is not an allergy or an intolerance to gluten.

Diagnosis:

Screening for coeliac disease involves:

- serology: to screen for coeliac disease
- tTg (tissue transglutaminase)
- anti-endomysial antibodies.

It is important to check IgA levels. Tissue transglutaminase antibodies are an IgA subclass and if the IgA level is low then the test can be a false -ve.

A duodenal biopsy to confirm the diagnosis is the the gold standard.

Testing is also recommended if the patient has any of the following conditions:

- type 1 diabetes
- irritable bowel syndrome (IBS)
- under or overactive thyroid glands
- dermatitis herpetiformis.

Complete gluten avoidance is necessary and eating even tiny amounts can trigger symptoms of coeliac disease and increase the risk of developing the following complications:

- osteoporosis
- malnutrition
- infertility
- malignancy – there is an increased risk of developing lymphomas.

Foods containing gluten include:

- bread
- pasta
- cereals
- biscuits or crackers
- cakes and pastries
- pies
- gravies and sauces.

For more information, see:

http://www.nhs.uk/conditions/Coeliac-disease/Pages/Introduction.aspx

http://www.nice.org.uk/nicemedia/pdf/CG86FullGuideline.pdf

http://www.nhsdirect.wales.nhs.uk/encyclopaedia/c/article/coeliacdisease/

For your notes and thoughts

Data interpretation station: case 5

Hyperthyroidism

Information given to the candidate

Kerry, a 12-year-old girl, is referred by her school nurse with a poor attention span and hyperactivity over the last few months. She has lost some weight despite having an increased appetite. During games she tends to sweat more than before.

Your task

Please review the information below.

You have two minutes to analyse the data and then four minutes to discuss your interpretation and management, if appropriate, with the examiner.

Data provided

Hb	13.6 g/dl – 136g/L
WBC	8.4×10^9/L
Neutrophils	6.6×10^9/L
Lymphocyte	1.7×10^9/L
Platelets	418×10^9/L
Sodium	140 mmol/L
Potassium	4.2 mmol/L
Urea	4.5 mmol/l
CRP	2 mg/L
TSH	0.03 miu/L (0.1 – 5)
Free T$_4$	62.5 pmol/L (9-24)
Free T$_3$	39.6 pmol/L (3.8-7)
Anti TPO antibodies	95 iu/mL (0-35)
ALT	25 U/L (8 - 40 U/L)
AST	21 U/L (15–50)

Questions

What are the abnormalities and what is your working diagnosis?

What would you do?

What advice will you give Kerry and her parents?

What is expected from the candidate

The candidate should:

- identify very low TSH with raised T3 and T4, indicating hyperthyroidism
- identify that increased antibodies suggest an autoimmune pathology
- be able to list a few features of the condition and the principles of management.

Answers

What are the abnormalities and what is your working diagnosis?

- Low TSH.
- High free T_4 and free T_3.
- Hyperthyroidism.

What would you do:

- Check for other signs, such as tachycardia, lid lag, tremor.
- Block 'production' of thyroxine from the thyroid. This management can be medical, initially – carbimazole.
- Consult paediatric endocrinologist for advice.

What advice will you give Kerry and her parents?

- Reassure them about the symptoms, signs and the diagnosis.
- Discuss treatment and the need for further opinions.
- Arrange for a follow up appointment/safety net.

For your notes and thoughts

Data interpretation station: case 6

Rickets

Information given to the candidate

Mohammad, a one-year-old boy, has recently moved to the UK. He is referred by a health visitor for further evaluation of poor growth. His birth history was uneventful and he was exclusively breast fed for eight months. On examination, both his height and weight are just below the 2nd centile and he has a prominence of the anterior costochondral junction. His systemic examination was otherwise essentially normal.

Your task

Please see the information below.

You have two minutes to analyse the data and then four minutes to discuss your interpretation and management, if appropriate, with the examiner.

Data provided

Hb	8.6 g/dl – 86g/L
WBC	8.9×10^9/L
Neutrophils	6.2×10^9/L
Lymphocyte	1.7×10^9/L
Platelets	196×10^9/L
Sodium	139 mmol/l
Potassium	4.2 mmol/l
Urea	3.5 mmol/l
Creatinine	36 umol/l
Corrected Ca	1.7 mmol/l (2.1 – 2.7)
Phosphate	0.46 mmol/l (1.0 – 1.8)
Alkaline phosphate	2346 u/L (117- 500)
Coeliac screen	Negative
Sweat test	Negative

Questions

What are the abnormalities and what is your working diagnosis?

What would you do?

What advice will you give Mohammad's parents?

What is expected from the candidate

The candidate should:

- identify that prolonged, exclusive breast feeding can lead to nutritional deficiencies
- identify Mohammad's short stature and prominent rib cage – rickety rosary
- identify that calcium and phosphate are both low
- notice that there is markedly elevated alkaline phosphate – implying bone pathology.

Answers

What are the abnormalities and what is your working diagnosis?

- Low haemoglobin.
- Low calcium, phosphate, high alkaline phosphatase.
- Negative coeliac screen.
- Rickets – most likely to be nutritional.

What would you do?

- Perform x-rays of wrists, legs and chest to look for widening and cupping of metaphyseal region, splaying, fraying and generalised osteopaenia.
- Prescribe vitamin D supplement.
- Provide general nutrition advice and refer to a dietitian.
- Check other siblings.
- Arrange for review with dietitian.

What advice would you give Mohammad's parents?

- Explain the disease and its patho-physiology.
- Reassure them and explain that it is easily treatable with supplements.

Further information

The most common cause of rickets is a lack of vitamin D and calcium. In rare cases, children can be born with a genetic form of rickets. It can also develop if another condition affects how vitamins and minerals are absorbed by the body, leading to poor mineralisation of growth plates. It is only found in growing children.

There has been an increase in cases of rickets in the UK in recent years. Children of Asian, African-Caribbean and Middle Eastern origin have a higher risk because their skin is darker and they need more sunlight to produce enough vitamin D.

Clinical features:

- Craniotabes – early infancy.
- Frontal bossing and delayed closure of fontanelles.
- Widening of wrists.
- Delayed teeth eruption, extensive caries.
- Rickety rosary – enlargement of costochondral junction.
- Harrison groove.
- Pectus carinatum.
- Lumbar lordosis.
- Kyphoscoliosis, short stature.
- Bowing of legs – older children.

Investigations:

- Serum Ca/Phosphate.
- Alkaline phosphatase – always high if untreated.
- X-ray of wrists/knees.
- Renal functions.

Treatment options:

- Vit D (Caciferol/Ergocalciferol) ~ Vitamin D deficient types + Ca orally.
- 1α hydroxyD3 (Alfacalcidol).
- 125 (OH)2 D3 (Calcitriol).

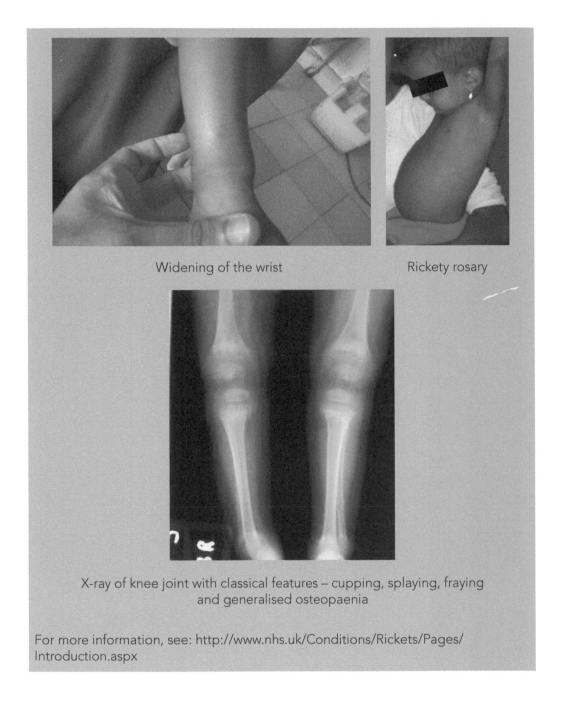

Widening of the wrist

Rickety rosary

X-ray of knee joint with classical features – cupping, splaying, fraying and generalised osteopaenia

For more information, see: http://www.nhs.uk/Conditions/Rickets/Pages/Introduction.aspx

For your notes and thoughts

Data interpretation station: case 7

Heart block

Information given to the candidate

Charlie, 12 years old, has comes to the clinic with his mother. He has a history of excessive tiredness and has been unable to attend school for the past two weeks.

Your task

Please see the information below.

You have two minutes to analyse the data and then four minutes to discuss your interpretation and management, if appropriate, with the examiner.

Data provided

Charlie has had an ECG done:

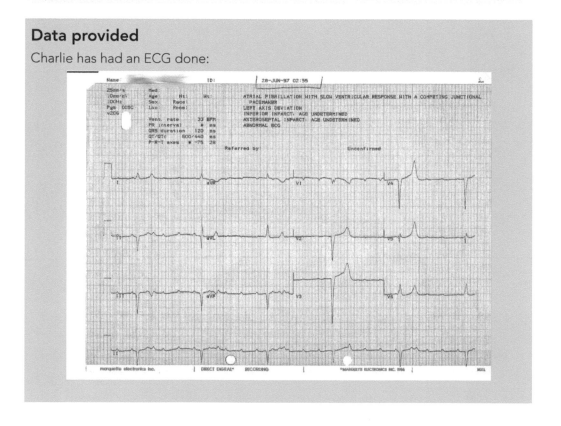

Questions

What are the abnormalities and what is your working diagnosis?

What would you do?

What advice will you give Charlie and his parents?

What is expected from the candidate

The candidate should:

- identify the data correctly
- pick up rate and rhythm on the ECG
- identify complete heart block
- identify P waves and independent QRS complex
- identify slow heart rate
- recognise that symptoms are due to slow heart rate
- diagnose congestive heart failure
- identify causes as: post-surgery, SLE, or rarely mitochondrial cardio-myopathy
- prescribe cardiac pacing as treatment.

Answers

What are the abnormalities and what is your working diagnosis?

- Slow heart rate.
- Dissociation of p wave and QRS.
- Complete heart block.

What would you do?

- Admit to hospital.
- Explain that a pacemaker will be required.

What advice will you give Charlie and his parents?

- Reassure them and explain the diagnosis.
- Explain management.
- Explain the reason for admission to hospital.

Further information

Acquired third degree heart block

The symptoms of acquired third degree heart block are:

- light-headedness
- dizziness
- fainting
- fatigue
- chest pain
- slow heart beat (bradycardia).

Heart block can be caused by several conditions and certain medications. It can be congenital or acquired.

Congenital third degree heart block cases develop in babies of mothers who have an autoimmune condition, such as systemic lupus erythematosis.

A number of medications can also cause third degree heart block, including:

- digoxin
- calcium-channel blockers
- beta blockers
- tricyclic
- clonidine – used to treat hypertensive crisis.

Heart block is diagnosed with an Electrocardiogram (ECG). Transcutaneous pacing (TCP) or temporary transvenous pacing (TTP) are short-term treatments of choice for symptomatic heart block.

For more information, see: http://www.nhs.uk/conditions/Heart-block/Pages/Introduction.aspx

For your notes and thoughts

Data interpretation station: case 8

Supra ventricular tachycardia

Information given to the candidate

Oliver is six months old and has been brought in as he is restless and not feeding.

Your task

Please see the information provided below.

You have two minutes to analyse the data and then four minutes to discuss your interpretation and management, if appropriate, with the examiner.

Data provided

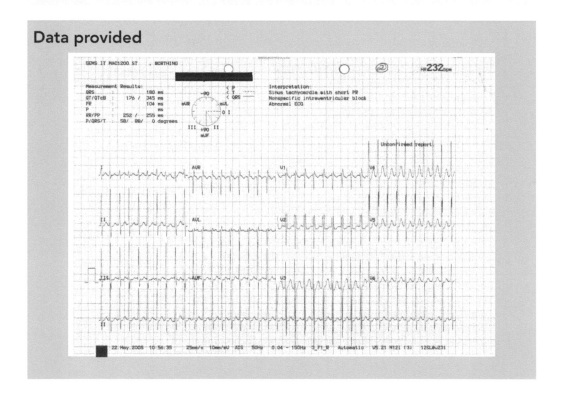

Questions

What are the abnormalities and what is your working diagnosis?

What would you do?

What advice will you give Oliver's parents?

What is expected from the candidate

The candidate:

- can diagnose the abnormality on ECG
- knows presenting symptoms
- understands management
- checks for cardiac decompensation
- does not alarm parents.

Answers

What are the abnormalities and what is your working diagnosis?

- Tachycardia.
- Narrow complexes.
- Supra ventricular tachycardia.

What would you do?

- Refer Oliver to the hospital urgently.
- Can try single carotid massage.
- Do not do ocular compression.

What advice would you give Oliver's parents?

- Explain that it is a common arrhythmia in children.
- No harm in the short term – children may be fractious – heart rapid but poor function.
- Explain that Oliver will need specialist care – WPW syndrome on resting ECG likely.

Further information

In supra ventricular tachycardia (SVT) the heart suddenly starts racing, then slows down abruptly. Episodes can last for seconds, minutes, hours or even days. They may occur regularly, several times a day, or very infrequently, once or twice a year. During an episode the heart rate may be as high as 250 beats per minute in infants, and up to 180bpm in children (a normal heartbeat should be 60–100 beats per minute at rest).

The symptoms include:

- irritability in infants
- racing heart
- chest pain
- dizziness/fainting
- light-headedness
- fatigue (tiredness)
- breathlessness.

Paroxysmal SVT is usually caused by a short circuit in the electrical system of the heart, which causes an electrical signal to travel rapidly and continuously around in a circle, forcing the heart to beat each time it completes the circuit.

In Wolff-Parkinson-White syndrome, an abnormal electrical connection occurs between atria and ventricles.

In many cases, SVT terminates spontaneously without treatment.

If acute treatment is needed:

- adenosine is injected as a bolus with flush so as to reach the heart relatively undiluted
- verapamil.

Medication may be also prescribed to prevent further episodes of SVT, including:

- flecainide
- beta blockers.

Cardioversion is occasionally used to stop an episode of SVT if there is evidence of decompensation.

Catheter ablation is an extremely effective procedure that 'burns' the abnormal tissue in the heart, thus blocking the abnormal electrical signal. Care must be taken not to damage the normal AV node.

For more information, see: http://www.nhs.uk/conditions/supraventricular-tachycardia/pages/introduction.aspx

For your notes and thoughts

Data interpretation station: case 9

Obstructive uropathy

Information given to the candidate

A test has been performed on Mark, an 18-month-old boy with recurrent urinary tract infections. His growth is normal and he is currently asymptomatic.

Your task

Please see the information provided below.

You have two minutes to analyse the data and then four minutes to discuss your interpretation and management, if appropriate, with the examiner.

Data provided

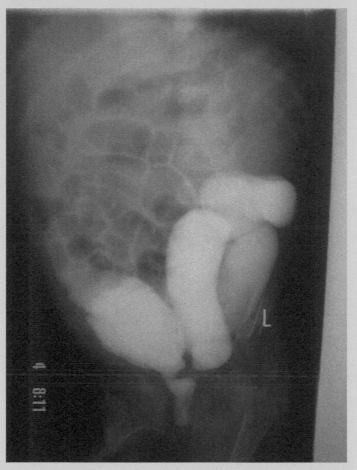

Questions

What is the test, the abnormalities and your working diagnosis?

What would you do?

What advice will you give Mark's parents?

What is expected from the candidate

The candidate should:

- be familiar with different types of renal imaging in children
- have basic interpretation skills to analyse the test results
- have an overall idea about the management of renal problems in children.

Answers

What is the test, the abnormalities and your working diagnosis?

- Micturating cystourethrogram (MCUG).
- Bilateral dilatation of ureters with vesico-ureteric reflux (VUR).
- Difficult to comment on the kidneys as they cannot be seen.
- Posterior urethral valves.

What would you do?

- Commence antibiotic prophylaxis.
- Refer urgently to paediatric surgeon/urologist.
- Monitor blood pressure and renal function.
- Regular monitoring of growth and other vital parameters.

What advice would you give Mark's parents?

- Explain the diagnosis and its effect on the kidneys.
- Explain the long-term implications of possible renal failure.
- Recommend a normal vaccination schedule.

Further information

Posterior urethral valve (PUV) disorder is the commonest urological cause of renal failure and subsequent renal transplantation in male children. Posterior urethral valves cause renal damage by causing back pressure.

This condition is only seen in males. An antenatal anomaly scan will show distended bladder and bilateral hydronephrosis.

Clinical features include:

- weak urinary stream and difficulty in micturation
- urinary tract infections
- palpable bladder, prune belly syndrome
- In later childhood – poor weight gain, secondary enuresis.

MCUG confirms the diagnosis.

Ablation of the valves is the definitive treatment, along with urinary prophylaxis for infections:

- 50% of patients will have VUR
- 30% will develop end-stage renal failure needing renal transplant.

For more information, see: http://www.nice.org.uk/nicemedia/live/11819/36030/36030.pdf

For your notes and thoughts

Data interpretation station: case 10

Polydipsia

Information given to the candidate

Sophie, a five-year-old girl, presented to the clinic with a history of secondary enuresis. Her mother gives a history of excessive thirst and passing large quantities of urine for the past three weeks. Her past medical history was unremarkable.

Your task

Review the information provided below.

You have two minutes to analyse the data and then four minutes to discuss your interpretation and management, if appropriate, with the examiner.

Data provided

Hb	12.3 g/dL – 123g/L
WBC	9.4×10^9/L
Neutrophils	8.0×10^9/L
Lymphocyte	1.3×10^9/L
Platelets	332×10^9/L
Sodium	138 mmol/L
Potassium	3.9 mmol/L
Urea	4.5 mmol/l
CRP	2 mg/L
Serum osmolality	286 mOsmol/kg H_2O (275 – 295)
Urine osmolality	245 mOsmol/kg H_2O (300-900)
Blood sugar	4.8 mmol/L (3.3 – 5.5)

Questions

What are the abnormalities and what is your working diagnosis?

What are the key investigations to confirm diagnosis?

What are the principles of management?

What advice will you give Sophie's parents?

What is expected from the candidate

The candidate should:

- have a basic idea of polydipsia and polyuria
- appreciate that serum osmolality is normal while urine osmolality is low
- identify that blood sugar is normal – thus it is not diabetes mellitus
- identify appropriate differential diagnosis
- discuss an appropriate management plan.

Answers

What are the abnormalities and your working diagnosis?

- Low urea, low/urine 245 mOsmol.
- Normal serum – 286 Osmol, normal blood sugar.
- Diabetes insipidus.
- Differential diagnoses:
  - diabetes mellitus.
  - psychogenic polydipsia.
  - chronic renal insufficiency.

What are the key investigations to confirm diagnosis?

- Three first urine samples, consecutive mornings, for urine osmolarity.
- Water deprivation test.

What are the principles of management?

- Fluid restriction.
- Behavioural therapy.

What advice will you give Sophie's parents?

- The condition psychogenic polydipsia can be treated and is not serious.
- Explain that Sophie will need to be referred to CAMHS.
- Try and restrict fluid intake and keep a record of drinking and passing urine.
- Follow up in out-patients.

Further information

Psychogenic polydipsia is a diagnosis by exclusion of other, more sinister pathologies. It is an uncommon condition seen in children often associated with compulsive behaviour and psychiatric disorders. It can be a symptom of emotional difficulties or an isolated feature in a child who simply enjoys drinking.

The excessive water drinking is well tolerated unless hyponatraemia occurs.

In chronic cases, hyponatraemia and water intoxication can occur. Severe hyponatraemia should be corrected to prevent neuropsychiatric complications such as confusion, seizures and delirium.

Diuretic therapy (Furosemide) may be beneficial in some patients as it preferentially causes water excretion over sodium excretion

A first morning specimen is the most concentrated sample a child will produce since during the night water intake should be minimal, hence three morning specimens of urine should be tested. If serum osmolality is <300 mOsmol/kg H_2O and urine osmolality is >600 mOsmol/kg H_2O urine/serum osmolality ratio >2, diabetes insipidus is excluded and further testing is unnecessary.

For more information, see:

http://www.gpnotebook.co.uk/simplepage.cfm?ID=-1999634384

http://www.ncbi.nlm.nih.gov/pubmed/17521521

For your notes and thoughts

Data interpretation station: case 11

Bilateral glue ear

Information given to the candidate

James is a seven-year-old boy who was referred as his teachers had noted a deterioration in his school performance.

Your task

Please review the information provided below.

You have two minutes to analyse the data and then four minutes to discuss your interpretation and management, if appropriate, with the examiner.

Data provided

This investigation is from a seven-year-old boy who was referred to you as his teachers had noted a deterioration in his school performance.

He was reviewed by an ENT specialist who conducted a hearing test. His audiogram is given below.

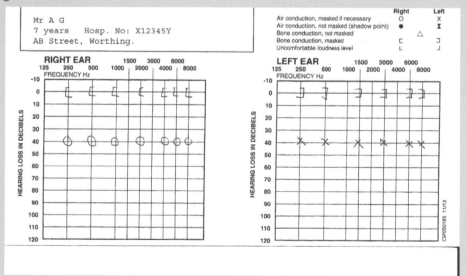

What is expected from the candidate

Diagnosis/differential diagnoses:

■ Bilateral conductive deafness

■ Bilateral serous otitis media

■ Bilateral glue ear.

Management plan:

■ Refer to ENT surgeon.

■ Inform school teacher.

■ Trial of treatment with antibiotics plus an antihistamine or nasal decongestant.

Further information

Chronic and varying hearing loss can significantly affect school performance and it is important to inform the school of a diagnosis. The teacher can then make appropriate adjustments such as sitting the child at the front of the class.

■ Up to 20dB loss does not cause noticeable problems with hearing normal conversation.

■ 20-40dB loss leads to conversation being heard as a whisper.

■ 40-60dB loss causes difficulty hearing loud speech ie. a teacher talking in a classroom.

■ 60-80dB loss leads to difficulty in hearing loud voices – which may, even then, not be understood.

Practical management will be to try a six-week course of antibiotics and nasal decongestants plus antihistamines while waiting for ENT review. If not resolved, the child will need grommets.

For your notes and thoughts

Structured oral station

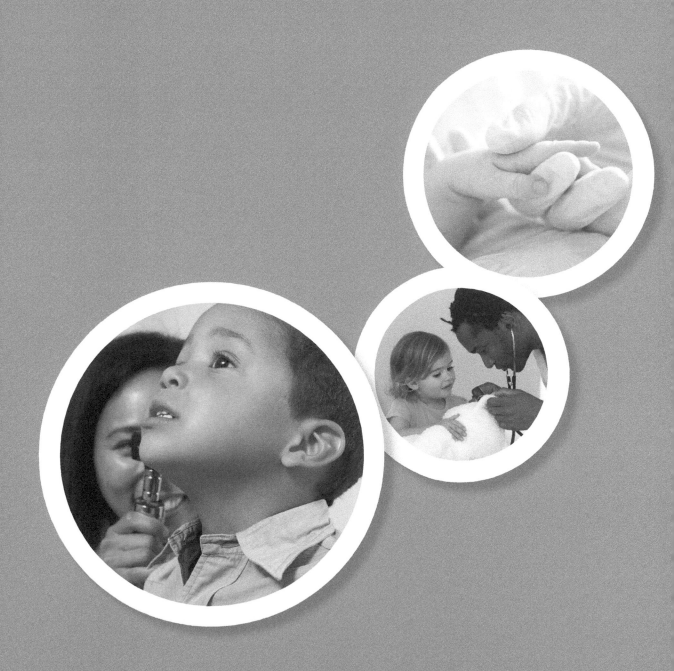

Structured oral station

The structured oral station is a new addition to the DCH examination. It is similar to a 'viva/interview', which you may be familiar with.

The station lasts six minutes. Before entering the exam room you will be provided with some information and given two minutes to digest it while you wait to be called in. When the examiner invites you in you will have some time to settle in and gather your thoughts together.

Each candidate will be asked the same questions, usually in the same order, but follow on questions can vary depending on the replies that you give. The discussion is usually based on your differential diagnosis and management of the clinical scenario given.

You will have enough time to answer the questions put to you and the examiner will normally not interrupt. As with all the stations, it is important that you ensure you fully understand the question so as to stay on track. If you do not understand the question, ask for a clarification. Think for a few seconds before you start speaking as that will reduce the 'umms and aahs'.

It is important that you are ready to support any judgements with the evidence provided, for example, 'I think the child has a non-accidental injury as the bruising is inconsistent with a fall from a small height on to a carpeted floor, the delay in presentation and inconsistent history'. This will allow you to move on to the next question and score better marks than if that information came out piece meal.

Keep a mental 'look out' for the five-minute warning as there will only be a minute left and you will need to summarise your answer, and you don't want to be left halfway through a sentence.

The examiner will be focusing on your reply and marking according to the guidelines discussed before the start of the examination session.

You can practise by making an audio recording or a video of your practice session with a friend in order to review and improve your 'performance'. Observe your body language, your speech, and the things you did not intend to say. I can reassure you that with practice you will improve your performance and this will be an asset at all the stations in the examination.

In this section we have supplied common questions after the clinical scenarios. We suggest you work with a colleague who can act as the examiner. However, if working alone, you should write down your thoughts after reading the scenario and use the answers provided as a guide. We have also added some relevant information at the end of the scenarios. Further information is available in the appendix, which will be useful in understanding the topics addressed in the scenarios.

Structured oral station: case 1

Non-accidental injury

Information given to the candidate

You are a GP. You have just seen Adam, a four-week-old baby with his mother referred by his health visitor. You note he has a large, boggy swelling on the back of his head, and dark-brown-bluish bruising on his anterior chest wall and abdomen. He lives with his mother and her boyfriend, John. She says Adam is a very active baby and rolled out of the bed on to a carpeted floor while she was in the kitchen.

Your task

You need to discuss the differential diagnosis and management with the examiner.

You have six minutes to complete the station; a warning bell will be given at five minutes.

Questions

What is your working diagnosis?

What would you do?

What advice will you give Adam's parents?

What is expected from the candidate

The candidate should:

- introduce themself to examiner
- provide fluent and structured answers
- explain in clear and simple language
- gather other relevant information ie. about the boyfriend
- reach a differential diagnosis with non-accidental injury (NAI):
  - Adam's injuries are not compatible with degree of fall/trauma described.
  - It is not possible for a four-week-old baby to roll off a bed.
  - He has suffered multiple injuries.
- explain that Adam needs to be seen at hospital for investigations
- not apportion blame
- understand that the situation may need social services input following hospital review.

Answers

What is your working diagnosis?

- Non-accidental injury.
- Accidental injury, but you are not being told the truth.

What would you do?

- Examine Adam fully and make detailed notes.
- Check history and make a note of what is described.
- Arrange for Adam to be seen urgently by local paediatrician.

What advice will you give Adam's parents?

- You are concerned about Adam's injuries.
- You are not convinced that the history given is compatible with his injuries.
- You will refer Adam to the local hospital for urgent review and investigations.

Further information

Child maltreatment includes:

- physical neglect ie. not properly caring for or looking after a child
- physical abuse ie. trauma
- emotional abuse
- sexual abuse
- fabricated or induced illness.

Follow local child protection guidelines on non-accidental injuries (NAI).

- Bruising is strongly related to mobility, and therefore bruising on a baby who is not mobile is very unusual.
- Abusive bruising often occurs on soft parts of the body such as the abdomen, back and buttocks.
- The head is the commonest site of bruising in NAI.
- Other common sites are the ears and neck.
- The age of an injury cannot be reliably estimated by the colour of the bruising.

The following investigations are mandatory in any case where physical abuse is suspected:

- A full skeletal survey – radiology of the whole skeleton to look for old or undiagnosed fractures.
- Clotting function, including full blood count for platelets.
- Biochemistry, including bone biochemistry.
- Appropriate investigations of the head if indicated ie. CT or MRI scans.
- Medical photography of any affected area.
- X-rays should be repeated after two weeks to check for callus formation on ribs.

Any history taken should include the dates and times of all events, and any inconsistencies should be recorded.

Good note-keeping is essential – dates and times, clarity, people present, signatures and designation. The notes in cases of NAI are more likely than any other to appear in court.

Black or blue ink should be used in case they need photocopying.

Any physical findings should be described in detail and a body map should be completed.

Clinical photographs, taken at the time, provide important information. Photographs should be taken early as bruises in children fade quickly.

Junior staff should try to avoid drawing inferences from findings, such as recording, 'Consistent with a gripping hand' – leave it to the senior member of the team.

For more information, see:

http://www.nspcc.org.uk/inform/research/findings/bruisesonchildren_wda48277.html

http://www.nspcc.org.uk/Inform/publications/downloads/bruisesonchildren_wdf48018.pdf

http://www.gpnotebook.co.uk/simplepage.cfm?ID=2006581296

http://publications.nice.org.uk/when-to-suspect-child-maltreatment-cg89

For your notes and thoughts

Structured oral station: case 2:

Chickenpox/shingles

Information given to the candidate

You are a GP and you are seeing Michael, a five-year-old boy, with his mother Susan. Michael has had a temperature and a runny nose for five days and has developed a rash with vesicles on the trunk in the last 24 hours.

Your task

You need to discuss your differential diagnosis and management with the examiner.

You have six minutes to complete the station; a warning bell will be given at five minutes.

Questions

What is your working diagnosis?

What would you do?

What advice will you give Susan?

What is expected from the candidate

The candidate should:

- introduce themself to the examiner
- provide fluent and structured answers
- explain in clear and simple language.

Answers

What is your working diagnosis?

- Chickenpox.
- Viral illness.
- Herpes/shingles.

What would you do?

- Explain the possibility of the illness being chickenpox. Generally, chickenpox is a mild illness in children but it can become secondarily infected and require antibiotic treatment.

- Check that Michael's mother is 'immune' to chickenpox and is not pregnant. Advise accordingly.

- Arrange to review Michael by home visit/phone consultation.

What advice will you give Susan?

- Keep Michael comfortable with regular paracetamol and plenty of fluids to drink.

- Give Michael antihistamines or topical creams if he is very itchy.

- Keep Michael away from public areas to avoid contact with people who have not had chickenpox.

- Keep him away from newborn babies, pregnant women and anyone who is immunocompromised.

Further information

At some point in their lives most children will contract chickenpox. It is a mild and common illness that causes a red rash of itchy spots that progress to fluid-filled blisters before crusting over into scabs and then eventually dropping off. These spots can sometimes cover the entire body, however some children will only develop a few. They are most likely to appear on the face and scalp, the ears, on and under the arms, on the legs and on the belly and chest.

90% of adults are immune to the condition because they have had it before. Chickenpox occurs in approximately three in every 1,000 pregnancies and can cause serious complications for both the pregnant woman and her unborn baby.

Complications include secondary bacterial infection, pneumonia, encephalitis, hepatitis, Reye syndrome, disseminated intravascular coagulation and post-infectious cerebellitis.

It is most infectious from one or two days before the rash appears until after all the blisters have crusted over, which is usually five or six days after the rash develops.

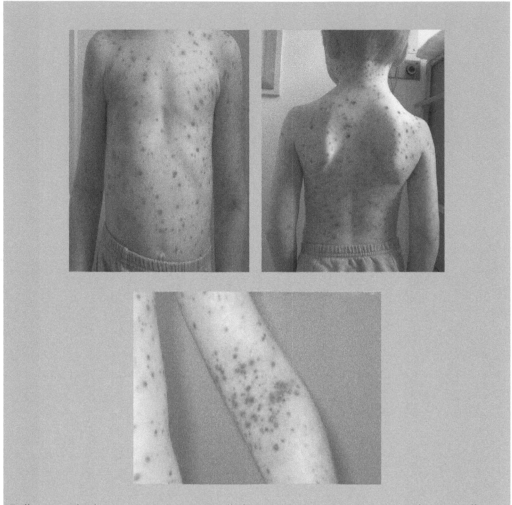

Following chickenpox, a person usually becomes immune. However, the varicella virus remains dormant in the body's nerve tissues and can return later in life as shingles.

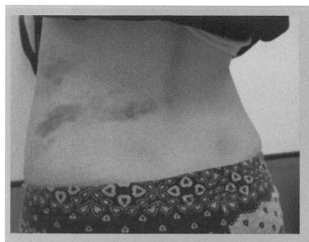

Shingles in an immuno-compromised patient on steroids

It is possible to catch chickenpox from someone with shingles, but not the other way around.

Although it is not part of the routine childhood vaccination schedule, there is a vaccine available. However, it is only offered to children and adults who may be susceptible to chickenpox complications.

For more information, see:

http://www.nhs.uk/Conditions/Chickenpox/Pages/Introduction.aspx

For your notes and thoughts

Structured oral station: case 3

Walking with a limp

Information given to the candidate

You are a paediatric SHO. Abdul, two years old, has been brought to the surgery by his mother for being fractious. You note he is walking with a limp and is unable to bear weight on his right leg.

Your task

You need to discuss the differential diagnosis and management with the examiner.

You have six minutes to complete the station; a warning bell will be given at five minutes.

Questions

What is your working diagnosis?

What would you do?

What advice will you give Abdul's parents?

What is expected from the candidate

The candidate should:

- introduce themself to the examiner
- provide fluent and structured answers
- explain in clear and simple language
- consider non-accidental Injury in their differential diagnosis
- safety net – follow-up.

Answers

What is your working diagnosis?

- Post-accidental trauma.
- Viral synovitis/arthritis.
- Non-accidental injury (NAI).

What would you do?

- Take a focused history of fall, infection.
- Examine for signs of infection – hips/knees/ankles.
- If concerned, discuss with senior or get a second opinion.

What advice would you give Abdul's parents?

- Depending on the cause, consider analgesia.
- Observe and follow up in 24–48 hours.
- Answer any concerns Abdul's parents have.

Further information

Limping can occur in children due to many reasons:

- Infections – septic arthritis/osteomyelitis
- Trauma
- Viral arthritis/discitis or synovitis
- Chronic inflammation – juvenile idiopathic arthritis
- Rare causes – malignancies (leukaemia, bone tumours).

Careful and repeated clinical assessment is the key to diagnosis. Knee pain in children often comes from the hip and sometimes the spine or thigh, so these must be examined. As with any limping child, infection has to be ruled out, which is the most important diagnosis to exclude. It is also important to consider and exclude appendicitis.

A child who cannot bear their weight, until proven otherwise, has:

- an infection
- a fracture
- a slipped capital femoral epiphysis (SCFE).

A well child who can bear their weight and has a full range of movement on examination is unlikely to have:

- an infection
- Perthes' disease
- SCFE.

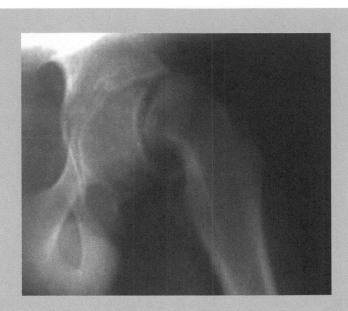

Slipped Capital Femoral Epiphysis requires urgent investigation and treatment. A typical presentation might be a teenager with groin pain after minor or no trauma and a reduced range of movement – typically flexion and internal rotation. An X-ray will be needed to exclude the diagnosis.

Perthes' disease is not an emergency, but it causes anxiety and so an outpatient appointment is needed as soon as possible.

An irritable hip – transient synovitis – is a diagnosis of exclusion and can only be made after X-rays, C-reactive protein, erythrocyte sedimentation rate and an ultrasound have helped in excluding a more sinister cause.

For your notes and thoughts

Structured oral station: case 4

Clavicle fracture in newborn

Information given to the candidate

You are a paediatric SHO. Adam is seven days old and has been referred by the health visitor because of a swelling noted over his left collar bone by his mother. On inspection you note a swelling over his left clavicle and, on palpation, note a mass 1cm in diameter. It is not particularly painful and Adam is moving both arms freely. He is otherwise breast feeding well, passing urine nicely, and his parents seem to be appropriately interacting with him. Adam weighs 4.95kg and had a difficult birth.

Your task

Please discuss your assessment, diagnosis and your management plan.

You have six minutes to complete the station; a warning bell will be given at five minutes.

Questions

What is your working diagnosis?

What would you do?

What advice will you give Adam's parents?

Diploma in Child Health: Volume 2 © Pavilion Publishing and Media Ltd and its licensors 2014.

What is expected from the candidate

The candidate should:

- introduce themself to the examiner
- provide fluent and structured answers
- explain in clear and simple language
- co-relate the history and physical examination findings to the commonest pathology of birth trauma
- ensure child safety (abuse) concerns are addressed
- provide a clear management plan and avoid unnecessary investigations.

Answers

What is your working diagnosis?

- This is likely to be a clavicle fracture sustained during delivery.
- The association includes:
  - humeral fracture
  - shoulder dislocation
  - brachial plexus injury.
- In case the lesion does not heal as expected, consider congenital pseudo-arthrosis of the clavicle. It may present as a newborn clavicle fracture and result from failed coalescence of the two primary ossification centres, which often presents late as a non-healing fracture.

What would you do?

- Examine (gently) the swelling over the clavicle, elicit crepitus if present.
- Ensure that the infant is clinically well and there are:
  - no other bruises
  - no torn oral frenulum.
- Enquire about the type of delivery and whether there was shoulder dystocia.
- Ensure that there are no child protection concerns (give a ring to social services) – rule out NAI.
- Consider organising an x-ray of the swelling (for medico-legal reasons as well as confirmation of the diagnosis).

What advice will you give Adam's parents?

- Reassure them that the clavicle fracture will heal spontaneously without any deformity.
- Provide advice regarding gentle handling and avoid pulling the baby by the arms.
- Educate his parents with regard to monitoring such fractures and give advice regarding healing time, which will help them in seeking medical advice where healing is delayed.

Further information

Clavicle fractures in newborns occur in 0.4–2.9% of all births.

Up to 40% of clavicle fractures may remain undetected at discharge (after newborn physical examination) from hospital.

They may also occur in uncomplicated and caesarean section deliveries.

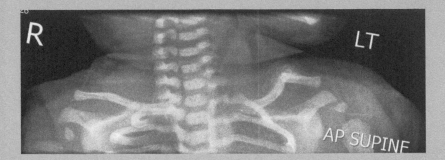

Concerns regarding child abuse/non-accidental injury (NAI) may arise in newborns with clavicle fractures, especially when such fractures are detected later as a callous formation or during an inter-current illness (eg. a chest X-ray done for respiratory illness).

Examination of the clavicle may reveal:

- crepitus
- palpable bony abnormality
- palpable spongy mass
- discoloration over the fracture site

In a study of 1,661 term newborns, a clinical diagnosis of clavicle fracture was made in 24 cases, 22 of which were confirmed by a radiograph or callous formation.

The most frequent clinical findings in a study of 22 children with clavicle fracture were:

- palpable spongy mass – 82%
- crepitus – 45%
- angulation deformity – 9%
- localised tenderness – 5%.

A clavicle fracture will heal spontaneously over a next few weeks with remodelling of the bone. No specific treatment is required. It is, however, important to follow up the patient to ensure adequate healing has taken place.

For more information, see:

http://radiopaedia.org/articles/birth-fracture-of-the-clavicle

http://www.ncbi.nlm.nih.gov/pubmed/9396889

For your notes and thoughts

Structured oral station: case 5

Febrile convulsion – talking to an anxious mother

Information given to the candidate

Aimee is two years old and has been unwell for two days. During the night she felt very warm to touch and had a seizure lasting one minute. She was seen by an out of hours doctor and was diagnosed with otitis media and a 'simple' febrile convulsion. Her father had 'fits' when he was young.

Your task

No further history is necessary.

Discuss the diagnosis and management with the examiner.

You have six minutes to complete the station; a warning bell will be given at five minutes.

Questions

What is your diagnosis?

Why did it happen?

What can be done about it?

What is expected from the candidate

The candidate should:

- introduce themself to the examiner
- provide fluent and structured answers
- have a good knowledge of symptoms, signs and differential diagnoses
- explain that febrile convulsion is not epilepsy and a simple febrile convulsion does not lead to brain damage
- also explain that one-third of children may suffer a subsequent febrile convulsion and the child should be laid down in recovery position. Do not insert anything in the mouth, and if lasts more than five minutes, call an ambulance; otherwise come to GP surgery for a check-up
- offer follow-up to review progress
- not use any medical jargon.

Answers

What is your diagnosis?

- With the history provided it is most likely that Aimee has otitis media and, due to her high temperature, had a seizure. There is enough information to make an informed judgement.
- Febrile convulsion secondary to infection – otitis media. They can be very frightening for parents, who think the child may die.

Why did it happen?

- Nobody is absolutely sure why it happens but in susceptible individuals (ie. those with a family history, with a sudden rise in temperature) there is a generalised tonic/clonic seizure. 10% to 20% of relatives have a seizure disorder.
- The seizure usually lasts between one and two minutes.
- The overall risk of further febrile seizures is one in three.

What can be done about it?

- In terms of immediate management it is important to rule out meningitis or other serious bacterial infection requiring treatment.
- A lumbar puncture should not be done on an unconscious child or with features of raised ICP.
- EEG is not indicated if the history and clinical findings are typical of febrile convulsion.
- Six per cent of febrile convulsions are prolonged and may be damaging, and should therefore be prevented.
- Advise parents to keep the child cool by removing warm clothing, tepid sponging and regular giving of paracetamol or ibuprofen.
- Prophylactic anti-epileptic medications are of no proven benefit and should not therefore be used.

Further information

- A febrile seizure/febrile convulsion occurs with a fever – fevers must be extra-cranial in origin.
- It may be the first indication to parents that a child is unwell.
- It is a relatively common childhood condition.
- During most seizures, the child's body becomes stiff, they lose consciousness and their arms and legs jerk. Some children may wet themselves.
- It may be tonic or tonic-clonic.
- Parents find the experience very frightening and often would say they thought the child was going to die.
- Most febrile seizures are harmless and do not pose a threat to a child's health.
- They can recur in about one-third of children in subsequent febrile illnesses.
- General advice is to keep the child cool and give antipyretics if required.
- During a fit, parents should observe basic life-support skills. These should be demonstrated to parents before discharging a child home.
- Long-term epilepsy incidence is the same as for general population, around one per cent.
- Antipyretics do not prevent febrile convulsions

For more information, visit: http://www.nhs.uk/Conditions/Febrile-convulsions/Pages/Introduction.aspx

For your notes and thoughts

Structured oral station: case 6

Painful legs – rhabdomyolysis

Information given to the candidate

You are a GP. You see Nicholas, 14 years old. He has severe pain in his legs, difficulty in walking and his urine has been pink/wine coloured for one day. He went for a 20-mile walk for a charity-sponsored function two days earlier.

Your task

You need to discuss the differential diagnosis and management with the examiner.

You have six minutes to complete the station; a warning bell will be given at five minutes.

Questions

What is your working diagnosis?

What would you do?

What advice will you give Nicholas and his parents?

What is expected from the candidate

The candidate should:

- introduce themself to examiner
- provide fluent and structured answers
- explain in clear and simple language
- identify the significance of his pink urine – negative for blood on testing
- admit a lack of knowledge and know when to seek help.

Answers

What is your working diagnosis?

- Post-traumatic muscle injury.
- Post-infectious myositis: coxsackie virus, influenza A virus and influenza B virus.
- Polymyositis, dermatomyositis.

What would you do?

- Confirm the diagnosis by:
  - testing urine for blood and myoglobin
  - testing blood: CPK levels – usually in >1,000 IU/L
  - testing blood: full blood count
  - testing renal function.
- Admit Nicholas to hospital and monitor urine output for signs of renal failure.
- Provide analgesia.

What advice will you give Nicholas and his parents?

- Explain the nature of the illness and the diagnosis.
- Bed rest, analgesics.
- Explain need for further specialist input.

Further information

Rhabdomyolysis is caused by muscle injury when muscle fibers break down and release their contents into the bloodstream. One of these released proteins, myoglobin, is harmful to the kidneys and may lead to kidney failure.

This can happen in extreme muscle strain in someone unused to strenuous exercise, but can also happen in trained athletes, especially marathon runners.

The following are common signs and symptoms of rhabdomyolysis:

- Myalgia – painful, swollen, bruised, or tenderness.
- Generalised weakness.
- Malaise, nausea and vomiting.
- Passage of dark urine (may have a low urine output).
- Extreme cases – confusion and impaired consciousness.

Common aetiological factors:

- Muscle trauma and crush injury.
- Infections – viral myositis.
- Extensive burns – muscle ischaemia.
- Excessive exertion – marathon, prolonged seizures.
- Metabolic conditions and congenital myopathies.
- Drugs and toxin mediated.

The most reliable test in the diagnosis of rhabdomyolysis is the level of creatine kinase (CPK) in the blood, usually >1,000 IU/L.

The urine, pink or red macroscopically, is 'negative' for blood on testing. The diagnosis is confirmed by presence of myoglobin in the urine plus high CK enzyme in blood.

The mainstay of treatment is generous quantities of intravenous fluids, but may include dialysis or hemofiltration in more severe cases.

For more information, see:

http://www.webmd.com/a-to-z-guides/rhabdomyolysis-symptoms-causes-treatments

http://en.wikipedia.org/wiki/Rhabdomyolysis

For your notes and thoughts

Structured oral station: case 7

Food allergy

Information given to the candidate

John is 22 months old and has come to see you with his mother, Jennifer. He developed a rash after eating a piece of bread with peanut butter. He has eczema and suffers from constipation. His mother has asthma and father suffers from hay fever.

Your task

You need to discuss the differential diagnosis and management with the examiner.

You have six minutes to complete the station; a warning bell will be given at five minutes.

Questions

What is your diagnosis?

Why did it happen?

What would you do?

What is expected from the candidate

The candidate should:

- introduce themself to the examiner
- provide fluent and structured answers
- demonstrate a good knowledge of symptoms, signs and differential diagnoses
- follow a systematic approach to get information
- ask about comorbidities
- know the correct investigations and their limitations
- understand appropriate management strategies
- explain in clear and simple language.

Answers

What is your diagnosis?

- With the history provided, it is most likely that John has had a reaction to something he has eaten.
- There is not enough information to make an informed judgement and some more information should be collected about:
  - how soon after eating the reaction occurred
  - where the rash was and its type
  - whether there was any associated breathing difficulties at the time.

Why did it happen?

- If the reaction was within a few minutes of John having eaten piece of bread with peanut butter, it is most likely to be a reaction to peanuts.
- Bread is unlikely to be the cause of the reaction.
- It could also be some other constituent in the peanut butter.

What would you do?

- The diagnosis needs to be confirmed by a skin-prick test or by measuring specific immunoglobulins (RAST).
- After the diagnosis is confirmed, you will:
  - explain to John's parents what has been found and what further needs to be done
  - provide an action plan, antihistamines and information leaflets/details of a support group
  - arrange for a dietitian review and follow up.

Diploma in Child Health: Volume 2 © Pavilion Publishing and Media Ltd and its licensors 2014.

Further information

History is the mainstay of diagnosis and management.

A food allergy is not the same as a food intolerance such as lactose intolerance and it is important to be aware of the distinction.

IgE mediated reactions are almost immediate and tend to occur in minutes rather than hours. Signs and symptoms include:

- pruritis
- erythema
- urticaria – localised or generalised
- angioedema – commonly of lips, eyes and face
- abdominal pain
- nasal itching, congestion, rhinitis and sneezing
- cough, chest tightness, wheeze or shortness of breath
- anaphylaxis.

Non-IgE mediated reactions, on the other hand, occur over hours or days.

During an examination, pay particular attention to:

- growth
- atopic eczema
- asthma
- allergic rhinitis
- signs of malnutrition.

Diagnosis

For IgE mediated reactions, skin prick tests (SPT) and/or specific IgE antibodies tests, previously known as RAST, should be used to check suspected foods that have been identified by the case history and the likely associated allergens.

SPTs should be carried out only at facilities equipped to deal with anaphylactic reactions. Do **not** do them in primary care settings unless necessary resuscitation facilities exist.

IgE mediated SPTs are affected by antihistamines but RASTs are not affected.

For non-IgE mediated reactions, eliminate suspected allergens for two to four weeks and then reintroduce after the trial.

Input from a dietitian will be required.

Do not use the following alternative diagnostic tools:

- hair analysis
- kinesiology
- VEGA test – measures electrical resistance with various allergens
- specific IgG to diagnose food allergy.

Lactose intolerance

Lactose intolerance is often confused with cow's milk protein allergy. It is due to a deficiency of the lactase enzyme, found in the brushfield border of the villi of small intestine epithelium. The commonest cause is damage to the epithelium following gastroenteritis. There is explosive, watery diarrhoea after ingestion of milk. The best management is avoidance of the lactose present in milk by giving lactose free milk – various formulae are available (SMA LF, Pregestamil – also partially hydrolysed). A lactose free diet should be followed for six to eight weeks in order for the brushfield border to repair itself, followed by the gradual reintroduction of normal milk.

For more information, see http://guidance.nice.org.uk/CG116

For your notes and thoughts

Structured oral station: case 8

Plagiocephaly

Information given to the candidate

You are a GP. You are reviewing Samuel, four months old, with his mother, Sandra. She is concerned about the shape of Samuel's head and is worried about his brain development in the future. She has seen a friend's son with a helmet.

You note Samuel to be well, showing normal development and a skull circumference 40cm. He has plagiocephaly.

Your task

You need to discuss the differential diagnosis and management with the examiner.

You have six minutes to complete the station; a warning bell will be given at five minutes.

Questions

What are your working diagnoses?

What would you do?

What advice would you give Samuel's parents?

What is expected from the candidate

The candidate should:

- introduce themself to the examiner
- provide fluent and structured answers
- explain in clear and simple language
- explain that plageocephaly is not pathological
- explain that it does improve with time
- explain that it is not associated with brain deformity or damage.

Answers

What are your working diagnoses?

- Plagiocephaly.
- Possible premature suture synostosis.

What would you do?

- Full general and developmental examination.
- Feeling of sutures and anterior fontanelle.

What advice will you give Samuel's parents?

- Reassure them that Samuel is developing normally.
- Plagiocephaly is a 'normal' variant in some children due to the position of the head.
- It will improve once the child starts moving his head and sitting – thus taking pressure off the occiput.
- There is no need for a helmet – they are expensive and have no long-term benefit in terms of development, although there may be some cosmetic difference.
- Explain simple measures that will allow active movement of his head to the opposite side.

Further information

Due to sleeping on their backs, a lot of babies develop a flattened head when they are a few months old. Often it will correct itself given time, and reassurance is all that is required. It develops because a baby's skull is still soft enough that constant pressure on one area can affect its shape.

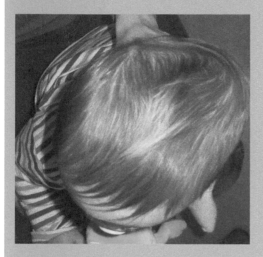

It is important for babies to sleep on their back as this reduces the risk of sudden infant death syndrome (SIDS). Change baby's position during the day to take some pressure off the flattened area.

For more information, see http://www.nhs.uk/conditions/plagiocephaly/Pages/Introduction.aspx

For your notes and thoughts

Structured oral station: case 9

Prolonged neonatal jaundice

Information given to the candidate

You are a GP registrar. A 15-day-old male infant, Jake, born at 38^{+6} weeks gestation with a birth weight of 3.56kg, has been brought to you as his mother is concerned that he looks yellow. The newborn screen showed normal results and the neonate has been exclusively breastfed from birth. His current weight is 3.75kg.

Your task

You need to discuss the differential diagnosis and management with the examiner.

You have six minutes to complete the station; a warning bell will be given at five minutes.

Questions

What are your working diagnoses?

What would you do?

What advice would you give Jake's parents?

What is expected from the candidate

The candidate should:

- introduce themself to the examiner
- provide fluent and structured answers
- demonstrate an understanding of prolonged neonatal jaundice and knowledge of the NICE guidelines for investigating such infants
- explain plans for further management by referring to local paediatricians for further investigations
- be aware of the need for objective assessment of an infant with prolonged neonatal jaundice (eg. weight gain, stool colour etc)
- arrange for follow-up to encourage the mother to continue breast feeding and discuss the investigation results (as parents are often informed that they will hear from the paediatric team if results are abnormal; otherwise their GP will be informed).

Answers

What is your working diagnosis?

- Prolonged neonatal jaundice.
- If the stool colour is normal, the child is breast feeding well and has been gaining weight, the most likely diagnosis in this scenario will be breast milk jaundice.

What would you do?

- Examine the infant to assess physical well-being and look for jaundice in natural daylight.
- Enquire about colour of stool and urine. If available, show the stool colour chart available from Children Liver Disease Foundation (www.yellowalert.org) for objective assessment of stool colour; see Figure 1.
- Refer to local paediatricians for organising blood and urine tests as per NICE guidelines.

What would you tell Jake's parents?

- Inform Jake's parents that he will need blood and urine tests at the hospital to find the cause of prolonged neonatal jaundice.
- Discuss the test results and encourage his mother to continue breast feeding.
- Explain that you will refer the neonate to a paediatrician for investigations.
- Arrange to see the infant a week later to find how they are doing.

Further information

Prolonged neonatal jaundice is a common presentation to primary care health professionals. It is therefore important that you have a good general understanding about the condition.

Jaundice is considered to be prolonged if a term baby (born at >37 weeks gestation) remains jaundiced at 14 days of postnatal life, or 21 days in the case of a preterm baby (born at <37 weeks gestation).

Most cases of prolonged neonatal jaundice in term infants are related to breast feeding, and is therefore called 'breast milk jaundice'. It is physiological, and breast feeding should NOT be discontinued. Mothers should be reassured and encouraged to continue to breast feed.

However, serious pathologies that can also present with prolonged jaundice in a neonate include:

- Unconjugated – infection (urinary tract infection), hypothyroidism, haemolytic anaemia (G6PD deficiency, spherocytosis)
- Conjugated – biliary atresia, metabolic conditions (galactosaemia).

It is important that clinicians are aware of the 'red flags' while assessing an infant with prolonged neonatal jaundice, when early referral should be considered:

Unwell baby with poor feeding and jaundice (may indicate sepsis, galactosaemia, UTI).

- Poor weight gain, coarse facies with jaundice (may indicate hypothyroidism).
- Pale stools and dark urine (using stool colour chart), may indicate biliary atresia).
- Significant jaundice on visual assessment may be associated with blood group incompatibility
- Parental concern about their baby being seriously unwell.
- Family history of inherited liver disorders eg. viral hepatitis B or C, Crigler-Najjar syndrome.

For more information on prolonged jaundice and to obtain your free information pack including the stool chart featured, contact Children's Liver Disease Foundation on 0121 121 6029 or email him@childliverdisease.org.

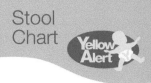

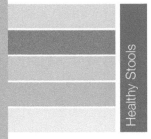

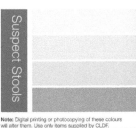

Stool Chart Yellow Alert

Healthy Stools

A healthy baby's stools can be any of these colours. Do not worry about green stools. Breast fed babies often pass watery stools. A sudden change to frequent watery stools of any colour may mean the baby is unwell.

- Breast-fed babies – often the stool colour is daffodil yellow
- Bottle-fed babies – often the stool colour is English mustard yellow

Suspect Stools

In babies with liver disease the stools may be one of the colours below. Do not worry about one or two stools that look unusual. Don't forget to look at the urine colour – in a new born baby it should be colourless.

Any baby with stools the colour below – whatever the age, should be investigated for liver disease.

Note: Digital printing or photocopying of these colours will alter them. Use only items supplied by CLDF.

Figure 1: Yellow Alert stool chart

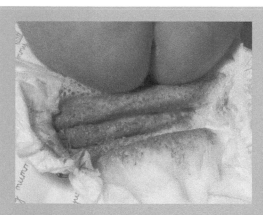 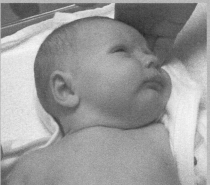

In term babies with a gestational age of 37 weeks or more with jaundice lasting more than 14 days, and in preterm babies with a gestational age of less than 37 weeks and jaundice lasting more than 21 days:

- look for pale chalky stools and/or dark urine that stains the nappy
- measure the conjugated bilirubin
- carry out a full blood count
- carry out a blood group determination (mother and baby) and DAT (Coombs' test) – interpret the result taking account of the strength of reaction, and whether the mother received prophylactic anti-D immunoglobulin during pregnancy
- carry out a urine culture
- ensure that routine neonatal screening (including screening for congenital hypothyroidism) has been performed.

(NICE Guidelines, CG98)

For more information, see: http://www.nice.org.uk/nicemedia/ live/12986/48680/48680.pdf

For your notes and thoughts

Structured oral station: case 10

Surgical emergency – strangulated inguinal hernia

Information given to the candidate

You are a GP registrar. You are seeing Henry, who is three months old, brought to you by his parents. He has been unsettled during the night, crying, refusing feeds and with some vomiting on two occasions. His parents have noticed a swelling in his groin for the past two months to be more firm and tense. There is no discoloration of the overlying skin. You note the swelling is tender and not particularly warm, and you cannot get above it, but you can feel the testes separately. The swelling does not trans-illuminate. He is passing urine nicely with a good stream.

Your impression is that Henry has a strangulated inguinal hernia.

Your task

Discuss your assessment, diagnosis and your management plan with the examiner.

You have six minutes to complete the station; a warning bell will be given at five minutes.

Questions

What is your working diagnosis?

What would you do?

What advice will you give Henry's parents?

What is expected from the candidate

The candidate should:

- introduce themself to examiner
- provide fluent and structured answers
- be able to pick up the pathology by co-relating it with the clinical history and the examination findings
- clearly explain the management plan to Henry's parents
- consider the need for surgery and advise to keep the child nil-by-mouth
- mention urgent referral to paediatricians/surgeons, realising that a strangulated inguinal hernia is a surgical emergency. Avoid unnecessary investigations.

Answers

What is your working diagnosis?

- It is a hernia because:
  - you cannot get over the swelling
  - the swelling does not trans-illuminate.
- This is likely to be a strangulated inguinal hernia as:
  - it is tender
  - cannot be reduced by gentle pressure when the child is relaxed
  - there is vomiting.
- The differential diagnosis would be a hydrocele (where it would be possible to get above the swelling and is likely to trans-illuminate).
- Need to consider infection locally that may cause lymphadenopathy or, rarely, malignancies.

What would you do?

- Examine the child to ensure he is otherwise systemically well and vital observations (pulse rate, respiratory rate, temperature, central capillary refill time) are stable (ABC).
- Refer urgently to the local paediatricians/surgeons with a clinical diagnosis of strangulated inguinal hernia.
- Administer pain relief if necessary.

What advice will you give Henry's parents?

- Inform Henry's parents that the swelling is an inguinal hernia that is likely to be obstructed. It is a surgical emergency.
- Inform them that you are going to refer Henry urgently to a paediatrician/surgeon and that an operation is likely to be required.
- Advise parents to keep the child nil-by-mouth in preparation for surgery.
- Offer the parents a review at the surgery in two weeks' time to know progress and/or monitor recovery post-surgery.

Further information

Surgical topics can be encountered in the DCH examination. Emergencies are more likely to be discussed and commonly seen conditions include:

- appendicitis
- intussusceptions
- strangulated inguinal hernias
- torsion of the testes
- intestinal obstruction.

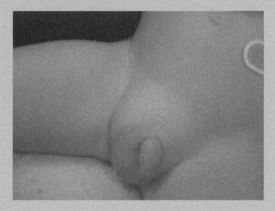

You will be expected to make these diagnoses and recommend an early referral to specialist services.

Bile stained vomit in a child is abnormal and is one of the most consistent signs of serious surgical pathology. This should trigger an urgent referral from primary care.

Indirect inguinal hernias have an increased incidence in premature infants. The formation of inguinal hernias in children is directly linked to descent of the developing gonads.

For more information, see: http://www.pediatricurologybook.com/inguinal_hernia.html

For your notes and thoughts

Safe prescribing station

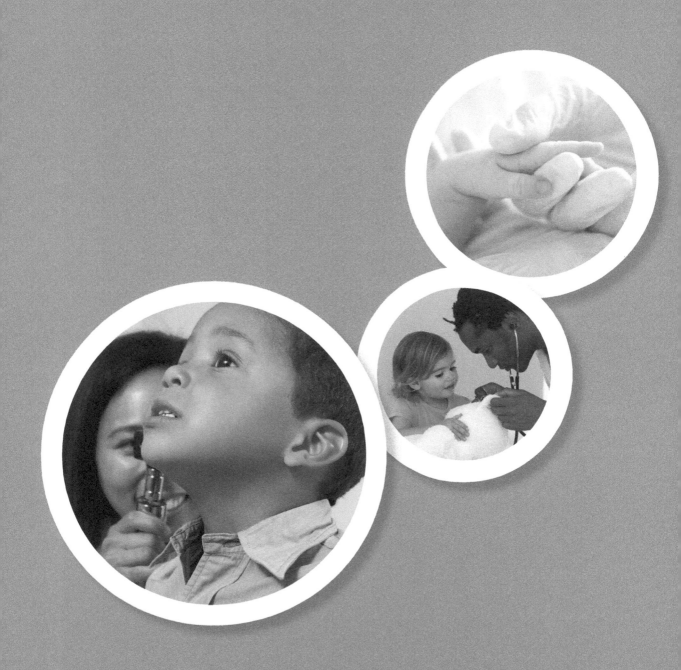

Safe prescribing station

The RCPCH has a dedicated station in the DCH examination to assess candidates' prescribing skills for commonly used drugs in paediatrics. This is due to the potential of harm to patients following a drug error.

In one definition, 'medication error' was described as 'a failure in the treatment process that leads to, or has the potential to lead to, harm to the patient' (Aronson, 2009).

Medication errors are among the most common medical mistakes and account for significant morbidity and mortality. In young adults (between 16–45 years) it is believed to be the second most common cause of death, after accidents.

Medication errors can occur at any one of three stages that a medication goes through:

1. Prescribing.
2. Dispensing.
3. Administration.

Reducing these errors is the single most effective way of reducing harm to patients.

In a four-week prospective study of 36,000 prescriptions in UK, 1.5% were found to have a prescribing error, 25% of which were potentially serious.

When only serious errors were examined, 58% of the errors were in the choice of the drug chosen and 42% were in the actual writing of the prescription.

Prescription errors are generally made by relatively junior doctors, who are often the first point of contact for patients and who tend to write the most prescriptions. The majority of these errors are not due to reckless behaviour on the part of prescribers, but rather the complexity of medication use in the highly technical environment in which we work (Williams, 2008).

Some of the errors commonly seen include:

- incomplete medication history ie. allergies or incomplete list of medications being taken with dosage

- incomplete patient details

- wrong choice of medication

- confusion over drug name

- lack of knowledge of prescribed drug

- inadequate knowledge of recommended use

- inadequate knowledge of recommended dosage

- lack of adequate knowledge of interactions between drugs

- lack of knowledge of contraindications

- incorrect use of decimal points leading to dosage errors

- abbreviations leading to confusion between various drugs

- illegible handwriting

- incomplete prescriber details

- inability to identify prescriber.

There have been great efforts made to reduce these drug errors and extra teaching and practice is provided to doctors to improve their knowledge of drug prescribing.

When writing a prescription, the following guidelines should be observed:

- The name of the patient should be clearly written. In addition, there should be two other pieces of identification:
  - date of birth
  - address
  - hospital or unit number.

- The date of prescribing should be clearly mentioned.

- In paediatric patients, it is good practice to write **both date of birth and weight** as most drug dosages are calculated on weight.

- Correct medication should be chosen as per common guidelines and practice.

- It is important to cross-check with history of allergy or other disease conditions such as the use of beta blockers with a history of asthma.

- Do not confuse similar sounding drugs.

- Check and confirm indication.
- Check contraindications before deciding on the drug.
- Check the dosage – the British National Formulary for Children (BNFC) gives detailed information on dosage:
  - Gaviscon is available in infant sachets that are equal to two doses.
  - confirm the frequency.
- Do not start on the maximum dose of a drug – generally titrate up depending on the response.
- A drug should be prescribed by generic name wherever possible.
- Use decimal points appropriately, as follows:
  - a zero should always precede a decimal point (eg. 0.5ml and not .5ml)
  - unnecessary use should be avoided (eg. 3mg and not 3.0mg)
- Use written mg/milligrams /micrograms:
  - quantities less than 1g should be written in milligrams (eg. 500mg and not 0.5g)
  - quantities less than 1mg should be written in micrograms (eg. 100 micrograms and not 0.1 mg).
- 'Micrograms' and 'nanograms' should **not** be abbreviated.
- Avoid using abbreviations for drug names (eg. AZT can be confused between azathioprine and zidovudine).
- Dose and frequency should be stated – in case of medications to be taken 'as required', **a minimum dose interval** should be prescribed.
- Oral liquid preparations: 'millilitre' (ml or mL) is used not cubic centimetre (cc), if not in multiples of 5ml an **oral syringe should be provided**.
- Suitable quantities should be mentioned:
  - paediatric mixtures (5ml dose) – 50, 100 or 150ml
  - lotions – 200ml
  - quantity supplied may be mentioned by writing the number of days of treatment required.
- Directions should be written in English without abbreviations but certain Latin abbreviations are accepted and used:
  - o.d.   –   omni die (every day)
  - b.d.   –   bis die (twice daily)
  - t.d.s   –   ter die sumendum (to be taken three times a day)
  - q.d.s   –   quater die sumendum (to be taken four times a day)

- ■ p.r.n – pro re nata (when required)
- ■ stat – immediately
- ■ o.n – omni nocte (every night)

- Check for side effects as you will be expected to discuss them with the patient/parent/examiner.

- Always include the signature of prescriber.

- Include the name of prescriber clearly written beneath the signature.

- The date should be clearly written.

- Include the address of prescriber/contact details in case there is a query from the dispensing chemist or nurse.

- Legible and clear handwriting is vital.

The FP10 prescription

The FP10 is a prescription used by GPs in the UK. In hospital settings, prescriptions are of a different format. However, legally, any paper with the correct and adequate information can be used as a prescription.

The following is a specimen of an FP10 prescription:

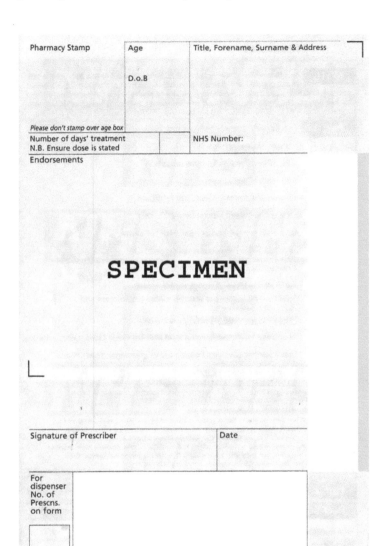

Any appropriate prescription may be used but it is essential to include all the relevant information.

The BNFC is the recommended source of drug, dosage and prescribing information for use in UK hospitals, and is in fact used by doctors in many other countries. It gives clear guidance on how to write a prescription, accepted abbreviations, the various drugs suitable for children, their indications, contraindications, side effects and interactions along with the cost.

Access to the BNFC is available for the prescribing station.

The station is assessed and marked on the following criteria:

Prescribing effectively and in context – first set of marks
Essential:

- Name, address, date of birth (weight – extra point).

- Correct drug.

- Generic name or trade name (if appropriate).

- Legibility.

- Correct dose:
    - 0 before a decimal point
    - dose strength
    - units clearly written: g, mg, microgram, nanogram.

- Dose frequency and total number of days of dose indicated.

- Signature.

- Name clearly written.

Desirable:

- Formulation – most suitable eg. liquid/capsule.

- Dispensable dose – rounded up.

- Appropriate route of administration.

- Weight of patient.

Knowledge, skills and attitude to prescribing – second set of marks

- Explains correct choice (clinical plus cost effectiveness):
    - clinical reasoning
    - national guidelines or BNFC advice.

- Explains the relevant patient-related factors influencing decision.

- Demonstrates knowledge of contraindications.

- Demonstrates knowledge of side-effects.

- Fluent and confident in discussion with the examiner.

Using this chapter

This chapter contains a series of scenarios providing you in the first box with some brief details of a case and some important information about the patient.

Once you have made a diagnosis, you will have four minutes to complete a prescription using the sample FP10 on p106. You will then have two minutes for discussion with the role player, following the questions in the second box, usually asking for your diagnosis and what you have prescribed, if there are any side effects and what further advice you would give to the patient or their parents.

Your study partner will have access to the third box, containing the 'answers' to these questions and an example of a 'correct' prescription.

We have included in this study guide many common conditions normally seen in primary care and we give examples of 'best practice' prescriptions and important information related to the drugs necessary for discussion with the examiner.

On the following page you will see the blank sample FP10 prescription. You should photocopy this page as many times as you need, so you have a clean example for each of the exercises.

In the examples, we recommend you write out the prescription under examination conditions, and then compare it with the 'answer' provided.

In the exam itself you will be given three minutes to read the scenario provided, and then invited into the examination room. There you will be provided with a blank FP10 prescription and a copy of the BNFC.

There are no patients at this station, so your study partner will be playing the role of the examiner, with whom you must discuss your diagnosis and your answers to the questions.

Remember, practice makes perfect.

References and further reading

Aronson J K (2009) Medical errors: what are they, how they happen, and how to avoid them. *QJM* **102** (8) 513–521.

Williams D J P (2007) Medication errors. *J R Coll Physicians Edinb* **37**:343–346

Available from:

http://www.rcpe.ac.uk/journal/issue/journal_37_4/Williams.pdf [accessed March 2014].

http://www8.nationalacademies.org/onpinews/newsitem.aspx?recordid=11623

http://www.nice.org.uk/mpc/index.jsp

Sample FP10

Pharmacy Stamp	Age	Title, Forename, Surname & Address
	D.o.B	
Please don't stamp over age box		NHS Number:

Number of days' treatment N.B. Ensure dose is stated		

Signature of Prescriber	Date

For Dispenser No. of Prescns. on form	

Safe prescribing station: case 1

Asthma

Information given to the candidate

Alex Broadgreen brings his four-year-old daughter, Anna, to the surgery. She is frequently wheezy and uses a salbutamol 100 microgram inhaler with a yellow aerochamber two or three times a week to relieve her symptoms. This has been going on for several months, however in the last two weeks her father reports that she has been coughing a lot at night.

Name: Anna Broadgreen

DOB: 27/08/2008

Address: 28B The Willows, Hollingdean, Brighton, BN9 4WS

Hospital/NHS No:

Weight: 17 kg

Your task

You need to write a prescription in four minutes and then discuss your prescription and choice of treatment with the examiner for two minutes.

You have six minutes to complete the station; a warning bell will be given at five minutes.

Using the sample FP10 on p106, please write the prescription as in the examination.

Questions

What is your working diagnosis and what have you prescribed?

What are the side effects?

What instructions or advice would you give Anna's parents?

What is expected from the candidate

The candidate should:

- introduce themself to the examiner
- provide fluent and structured answers
- write a clear and legible prescription
- choose an appropriate drug
- state the correct dose and the correct route of administration for the correct duration
- follow a systematic approach to get information from the BNFC
- demonstrate a knowledge of comorbidities, side effects, indications and contraindications
- explain in clear and simple language.

Answers

What is your working diagnosis and what have you prescribed?

- Asthma – not adequately controlled.
- Frequent use of salbutamol and night cough.
- **Prescription:** Beclometasone – prophylaxis for asthma.

What are the side effects?

- Hoarseness.
- Dysphonia.
- Adrenal suppression.

What instructions or advice would you give Anna's parents?

- The child should rinse their mouth or brush their teeth after each use.
- Regular use is important – even if she is not symptomatic.
- Use the salbutamol inhaler as needed and keep a record.

Copy of 'correct' prescription.

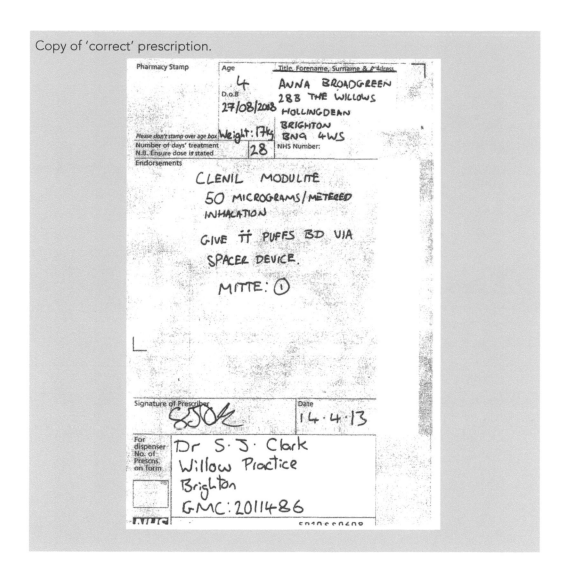

Further information

Beclometasone inhaler – given as a metered dose inhaler (MDI) to used with a spacer.

Indication: prophylaxis of asthma.

Cautions: high doses in children can lead to adrenal suppression.

Side effects: hoarseness, dysphonia and oral thrush.

Good prescribing points: The child should rinse out their mouth with water or brush their teeth after each use of the inhaler to prevent deposition of powder in the mouth, which can lead to oral thrush.

Beclometasone CFC-free pressurised metered-dose inhalers (QVAR and Clenil Modulite) are not interchangeable and should be prescribed by brand.

Parents should be advised that steroid inhalers need to be used regularly as they prevent exacerbations of asthma.

Clinical features that increase the probability of asthma include symptoms of wheeze, cough, difficulty breathing and chest tightness – particularly if these:

- are frequent and recurrent
- are worse at night and in the early morning
- occur in response to, or are worse after, exercise or other triggers.

Other clinical features that point to asthma are a personal or family history of atopic disorder, widespread wheeze of auscultation and a history of improvement in symptoms or lung function in response to adequate therapy.

It is important for candidates to be familiar with British Thoracic Society guidelines for asthma management.

For more information, see:

http://www.brit-thoracic.org.uk/Portals/0/Guidelines/AsthmaGuidelines/sign101%20Jan%202012.pdf

For your notes and thoughts

Safe prescribing station: case 2

Head lice

Information given to the candidate

Stacey Williams, a two-year-old girl, is brought to the surgery by her 30-year-old father, Chris, along with her brother, Jack, who is six. Both Stacey and Jack have been scratching their heads for a few days and their dad has found small white specks on the scalp at the back of the children's necks.

You diagnose them to have head lice. Stacey has recently been diagnosed with asthma.

Name: Stacey Williams
DOB: 17/11/2010
Address: 18 Shakespeare Road, Bedford, BD25 6PP
Hospital/NHS No: A12358C
Weight: 10 kg.

Your task

You need to write a prescription in four minutes and then discuss your prescription and choice of treatment with the examiner for two minutes.

You have six minutes to complete the station; a warning bell will be given at five minutes.

Using the sample FP10 on p106, please write the prescription as in the examination.

Questions

What is your working diagnosis and why have you chosen this prescription?
What are the side effects?
What instructions/advice would you give Stacey and Jack's parents?
Good prescribing points?

What is expected from the candidate

The candidate should:

- introduce themselves to the examiner
- provide fluent and structured answers
- write a clear and legible prescription
- choose an appropriate drug
- state the correct dose and the correct route of administration for the correct duration
- follow a systematic approach to get information from the BNFC
- demonstrate a knowledge of comorbidities, side effects, indications and contraindications
- explain in clear and simple language.

Answers

What is your working diagnosis and why have you chosen this prescription?

- Head lice.
- **Prescription:** Dimeticone 4% lotion.

What are the side effects?

- Skin irritation.

What instructions/advice would you give Stacey and Jack's parents?

- The infection can be transmitted to others.
- Rub the lotion into the scalp, leave for eight hours and rinse off.
- Repeat after seven days.
- Can also use a 'lice' comb.

Good prescribing points?

- Safe with children with asthma.
- As the patient has asthma, organophosphates such as malathion should not be prescribed.
- All family members should be treated.

Copy of a 'correct' prescription

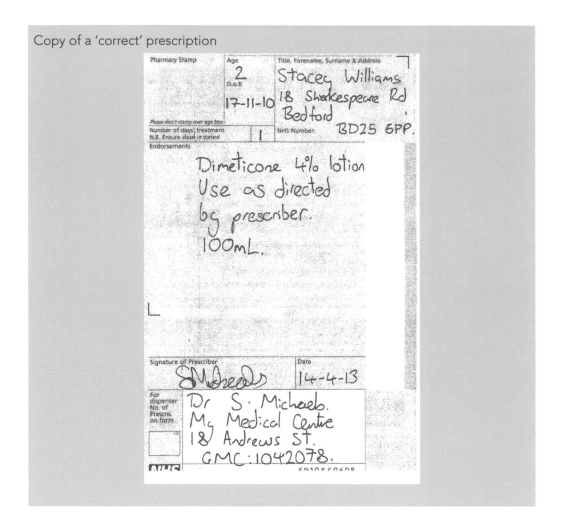

For your notes and thoughts

Safe prescribing station: case 3

Pain relief

Information given to the candidate

Michael Smith brings his 10-year-old son Billy to the surgery on Monday morning. Billy was playing football with his friends over the weekend and was 'kneed' in the right quadriceps during play. He has been limping and was therefore brought to surgery. Following examination, you are confident that the area is badly bruised but with only a little swelling.

Billy has no known drug allergies and no past medical history. Billy is very keen for you to make him better because he has a football match in two days for the school team.

Please advise Mr Smith on the best course of action and prescribe for Billy if you feel it is appropriate.

Name: Billy Smith

DOB: 12/03/2003

Address: 121 Edge Lane, Stretford, Manchester, M4 6KL

              Hospital/NHS No: A234567B

Weight: 34 kg

Your task

You need to write a prescription in four minutes and then discuss your prescription and choice of treatment with the examiner for two minutes.

You have six minutes to complete the station; a warning bell will be given at five minutes.

Using the sample FP10 on p106, please write the prescription as in the examination.

Questions

What is your working diagnosis and what have you prescribed?

What are the side effects?

What instructions or advice would you give Billy and his parents?

What is expected from the candidate

The candidate should:

- introduce themself to the examiner
- provide fluent and structured answers
- write a clear and legible prescription
- choose an appropriate drug
- state the correct dose and the correct route of administration for the correct duration
- follow a systematic approach to get information from the BNFC
- demonstrate a knowledge of comorbidities, side effects, indications and contraindications
- explain in clear and simple language.

Answers

What is your working diagnosis and what have you prescribed?

- Trauma following an accident during football practice.
- No major obvious underlying injury.
- **Prescription:** Ibuprofen for pain relief and anti-inflammatory effect.

What are the side effects?

- Hypersensitivity to NSAIDs.
- Can potentially worsen asthma.

What instructions or advice would you give Billy and his parents?

- Ibuprofen is commonly used in soft-tissue injuries.
- He could also use paracetamol if the pain is not controlled by one drug.
- Rest – allowing time for tissues to heal – Billy will have to sit out his football games for a few days.
- He should be encouraged to walk when possible as light exercise.
- Inflammation and bruising will subside gradually over next seven to 10 days.

Copy of 'correct' prescription.

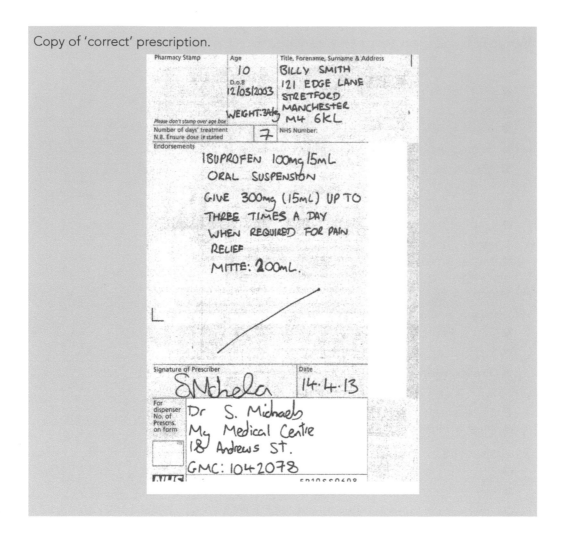

Pharmacy Stamp

Age
10

D.o.B
12/03/2003

WEIGHT: 34kg

Please don't stamp over age box

Number of days' treatment
N.B. Ensure dose is stated   7

Endorsements

Title, Forename, Surname & Address
BILLY SMITH
121 EDGE LANE
STRETFORD
MANCHESTER
M4 6KL

NHS Number:

IBUPROFEN 100mg/5mL
ORAL SUSPENSION

GIVE 300mg (15mL) UP TO
THREE TIMES A DAY
WHEN REQUIRED FOR PAIN
RELIEF
MITTE: 200mL.

Signature of Prescriber

Date
14.4.13

Dr S. Michaels
My Medical Centre
18 Andrews St.
GMC: 1042078

For dispenser
No. of
Prescns.
on form

For your notes and thoughts

Safe prescribing station: case 4

Eczema

Information given to the candidate

Martha Grayson brings her eight-month-old daughter, Emily, to the surgery. Emily has developed several patches of red, itchy skin over the past few weeks; one on her left cheek and in the folds of both her elbows. Emily has been admitted twice to hospital in past six months with episodes of wheezing.

Name: Emily Grayson
DOB: 13/09/2012
Address: 378 Marshall Avenue, Next Town, GY7 6TR
Hospital/NHS No: C234578A
Weight: 8.5 kg

Your task

You need to write a prescription in four minutes and then discuss your prescription and choice of treatment with the examiner for two minutes.

You have six minutes to complete the station; a warning bell will be given at five minutes.

Using the sample FP10 on p106, please write the prescription as in the examination.

Questions

What is your working diagnosis and what have you prescribed?

What are the side effects?

What instructions or advice would you give Emily's parents?

What is expected from the candidate

The candidate should:
- introduce themself to the examiner
- provide fluent and structured answers
- write a clear and legible prescription
- choose an appropriate drug
- state the correct dose and the correct route of administration for the correct duration
- follow a systematic approach to get information from the BNFC
- demonstrate a knowledge of comorbidities, side effects, indications and contraindications
- explain in clear and simple language.

Answers

What is your working diagnosis and what have you prescribed?
- Eczema with dry itchy skin.
- **Prescription:** Emollients.

What are the side effects?
- None.
- Short duration of effect, hence frequent use.

What instructions or advice would you give to Emily's parents?
- Eczema is a common condition in children. May be atopic.
- Needs regular moisturising.
- May be associated with certain allergies/sensitivities.
- If it does not respond or gets worse, the use of corticosteroids may be needed.

Copy of 'correct' prescription.

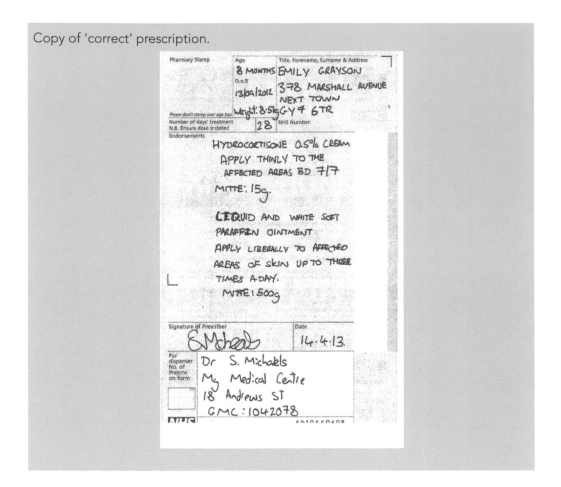

Further information

Emollients

Indication: dry skin

The effects of emollients are short-lived and they should therefore be applied frequently, even after an improvement in skin condition occurs. They should be applied immediately after washing or bathing to maximise the effect of skin hydration. Although light emollients such as aqueous cream are suitable for many dry skin conditions, greasier preparations such as white soft paraffin, emulsifying ointment and liquid and white soft paraffin ointment are often more effective.

Paraffin-based emollients in contact with clothes are easily ignited by a naked flame and therefore the patient's parent should be advised to wash their hands thoroughly after applying the emollient.

Corticosteroid

Indication: Inflammatory exacerbation of eczema.

Cautions: Avoid prolonged use of topical corticosteroids on the face.

Side effects: Although mild corticosteroids are associated with few side effects, the use of potent corticosteroids in infants can result in adrenal suppression from absorption through the skin.

To minimise the side effects of a topical corticosteroid, it is important to apply it thinly and to the affected areas only, no more than twice a day.

Further advice: Avoid irritation to the skin by avoiding extremes of temperature, dressing the child in non-abrasive clothing fabrics such as cotton, and reapplying emollients after wetting the skin.

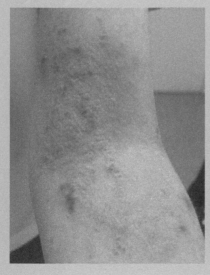 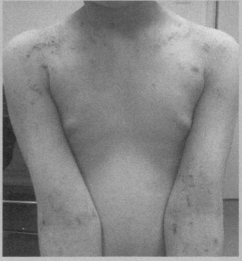

For your notes and thoughts

Safe prescribing station: case 5

Conjunctivitis

Information given to the candidate

Susan Jenkins brings her two-week-old son, Harvey, to see you with a sore right eye. It is red with crusty deposits on the lid margins. She has been cleaning it with warm water.

Name: Harvey Jenkins

DOB: 31/03/2013

Address: 6 Beachview, Worthing, BN11 2AB

Hospital/NHS No: A12357B

Weight: 3.5 kg.

Your task

You need to write a prescription in four minutes and then discuss your prescription and choice of treatment with the examiner for two minutes.

You have six minutes to complete the station; a warning bell will be given at five minutes.

Using the sample FP10 on p106, please write the prescription as in the examination.

Questions

What is your working diagnosis and what have you prescribed?

What are the side effects?

What instructions or advice would you give Harvey's mother?

Good prescribing points?

What is expected from the candidate

The candidate should:

- introduce themself to the examiner
- provide fluent and structured answers
- write a clear and legible prescription
- choose an appropriate drug
- state the correct dose and the correct route of administration for the correct duration
- follow a systematic approach to get information from BNFC
- demonstrate a knowledge of comorbidities, side effects, indications and contraindications
- explain in clear and simple language.

Answers

What is your working diagnosis and what have you prescribed?

- Conjunctivitis.
- Possible blocked nasolacrimal duct.
- **Prescription:** Chloramphenicol eye drops.

What are the side effects?

- Stinging on administration.

What instructions or advice would you give Harvey's parents?

- Practise good hand hygiene.
- Use eye drops as prescribed.
- The infection can be transmitted to others.

Good prescribing points?

- Supply one bottle of chloramphenicol for each eye.
- Continue eye drops for 48 hours after infection has resolved.
- Wash hands between administering drops into one eye before administering drops into the other eye.

Copy of a 'correct' prescription.

Pharmacy Stamp	Age D.o.B	Title, Forename, Surname & Address
	2 weeks Harvey Jenkins. 31/3/13.	6 Beachview Worthing BN11 2AB

Please don't stamp over age box

Number of days' treatment
N.B. Ensure dose is stated **7**

NHS Number:

Endorsements

Chloramphenicol 0.5%
eye drops.
↑ drop into Ⓛ + Ⓡ
eyes QDS until
48° after symptoms resolved.
2 bottles × 10mL.

Signature of Prescriber	Date
SMichaels.	14/4/13

For dispenser No. of Prescns. on form

Dr. S. Michaels
My Medical Centre
18 Andrew St.
GMC: 1042078.

Further information

Conjunctivitis is a very common eye infection.

Newborn babies are especially prone due to exposure during delivery.

In older children, the cause may be viral, bacterial or allergic.

The discharge is more noticeable first thing in the morning – crusting on eyelid at waking up.

The colour and consistency of discharge can aid in diagnosis:

- Bacterial conjunctivitis has a yellow discharge.
- Allergic conjunctivitis has a watery and clear discharge.
- Viral conjunctivitis has a sticky and clear discharge, almost always accompanied by flu-like symptoms.

A GP may take a swab of the discharge from the eye so that it can be tested for any bacteria or virus.

If there are a number of cases of conjunctivitis at one school or nursery, you might advise parents to keep their child away from the school until their infection has cleared up.

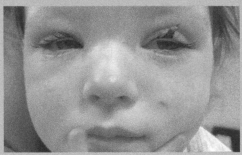

For more information, see:

http://www.nhs.uk/Conditions/Conjunctivitis-infective/Pages/Introduction.aspx

http://www.gosh.nhs.uk/medical-conditions/search-for-medical-conditions/conjunctivitis/conjunctivitis-information/

For your notes and thoughts

Safe prescribing station: case 6

Cow's milk protein allergy

Information given to the candidate

Claire is brought to see you by her mother. Claire is bottle fed, and for the past four weeks she has been very unsettled, vomiting and passing hard stools. You note that she has dry skin. Her mother is very distressed and upset.

Name: Claire Taylor

DOB: 24/02/2013

Address: 3 The Mews, Middleton, M24 4WS

Hospital/NHS No: A12356A

Weight: 4.5 kg.

Your task

You need to write a prescription in four minutes and then discuss your prescription and choice of treatment with the examiner for two minutes.

You have six minutes to complete the station; a warning bell will be given at five minutes.

Using the FP10 sample on p106, please write the prescription as in the examination.

Questions

What is your working diagnosis and what have you prescribed?

What are the side effects?

What instructions or advice would you give Claire's mother?

What is expected from the candidate

The candidate should:

- introduce themself to the examiner
- provide fluent and structured answers
- write a clear and legible prescription
- choose an appropriate drug
- state the correct dose and the correct route of administration for the correct duration
- follow a systematic approach to get information from the BNFC
- demonstrate a knowledge of comorbidities, side effects, indications and contraindications
- explain in clear and simple language.

Answers

What is your working diagnosis and what have you prescribed?

- Cow's milk protein allergy.
- Infantile colic/eczema.
- **Prescription:** hydrolysed milk – Nutramigen.

What are the side effects?

- None – although it is more expensive than normal milk.

What instructions or advice would you give Claire's parents?

- One scoop of powder to every 30ml of water.
- Bring Claire for review in two weeks.
- The benefits should be seen within 10–14 days.
- It should be given for up to one year in cases of cow's milk protein allergy.
- She may need further treatment with anti-reflux medication and emollients.

Copy of a 'correct' prescription.

Pharmacy Stamp	Age	Title, Forename, Surname & Address
	8 weeks D.o.B 24-2-13	Claire Taylor 3 The Mews, Middleton
Please don't stamp over age box		
Number of days' treatment N.B. Ensure dose is stated	28	NHS Number: M24 4WS
Endorsements		

Nutramigen 1
MDU.

2 tins
'ACBS'

Signature of Prescriber	Date
SMchola.	14.3.13

For dispenser No. of Prescns. on form

Dr S. Michaels
My Medical Centre
18 Andrews St.
GMC: 1042078

Further information

Breast feeding is the best, and is recommended exclusively for at least the first four months of life.

Five per cent to 15% of infants show symptoms suggestive of cow's milk protein allergy (CMPA). The prevalence of CMPA varies from two per cent to 7.5%.

CMPA is easily missed and should be considered as a cause of infant distress and diverse clinical symptoms including crying, vomiting, reflux, constipation and eczema.

CMPA persists in only a minority of children beyond two years of age.

It is to be differentiated from lactose intolerance or isolated GI tract infections.

Children with CMPA can present with a variety of clinical features that are cutaneous, GI, or respiratory in origin:

- Urticaria, atopic dermatitis, angioedema and contact rashes.
- Nausea, vomiting, haematemesis, colic, diarrhoea, occult and frank blood, enterocolitis, colitis, constipation and transient enteropathies.
- Rhinoconjuctivitis, asthma, wheezing, laryngeal oedema, otitis media and anaphylaxis

The prognosis depends on the child's age at presentation and titre of specific IgE to cow's milk protein at the time of diagnosis.

For more information, see:

http://adc.bmj.com/content/92/10/902.full

http://www.gpnotebook.co.uk/simplepage.cfm?ID=-268042236

For your notes and thoughts

Safe prescribing station: case 7

Meningococcal contact

Information given to the candidate

Daniel, a three-year-old boy, was admitted to hospital two days ago and has been confirmed to have meningococcal meningitis. A public health contact has asked you to provide prophylaxis for the family. He has an older brother.

Name: Michael Jones

DOB: 01/06/2006

Address: 71, Aldsworth Avenue, Another City, BN14 5JN

Hospital/NHS No: C234567A

Weight: 22 kg

Your task

You need to write a prescription in four minutes and then discuss your prescription and choice of treatment with the examiner for two minutes.

You have six minutes to complete the station; a warning bell will be given at five minutes.

Using the FP10 sample on p106, please write the prescription as in the examination.

Questions

What is your working diagnosis and what have you prescribed?

What are the side effects?

Safe prescribing points?

What instructions or advice would you give Daniel's parents?

What is expected from the candidate

The candidate should:

- introduce themself to the examiner
- provide fluent and structured answers
- write a clear and legible prescription
- choose an appropriate drug
- state the correct dose and the correct route of administration for the correct duration
- follow a systematic approach to get information from BNFC
- demonstrate a knowledge of comorbidities, side effects, indications and contraindications
- explain in clear and simple language
- mention other possible medications that may be used.

Answers

What is your working diagnosis and what have you prescribed?

- contact with meningococcal disease
- **Prescription:** Rifampicin.

What are the side effects?

- Rifampicin may cause:
  - orange-red discolouration of tears, urine and contact lenses
  - skin rashes and itching
  - gastrointestinal disturbance.

Safe prescribing points?

- It negates the effect of the oral contraceptive pill.
- It should not be used in pregnancy or in cases of severe liver disease.

What instructions or advice would you give Daniel's parents?

- Warn them about possible discolouration of urine, tears.
- Stress the importance of taking the full dose of medication.

Copy of 'correct' prescription.

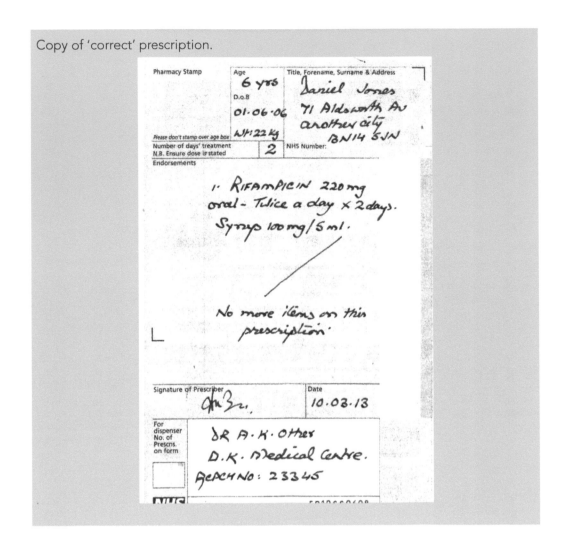

Further information

Meningococcal disease

Who requires prophlylaxis?

- Index case (if treated only with penicillin).
- All intimate, household or daycare contacts who have been exposed to index case within 10 days of onset.
- Any person who gave mouth-to-mouth resuscitation to the index case.

Drugs and doses:

- Rifampicin:
    - Adults: 600mg twice daily for two days.
    - Children: 10mg/kg twice daily for two days.
    - Neonates: 5mg/kg twice daily for two days.

Rifampicin may cause orange-red discolouration of tears, urine and contact lenses, skin rashes and itching, and gastrointestinal disturbance. It negates the effect of the oral contraceptive pill and should not be used in pregnancy or severe liver disease.

For pregnant women or if there is a contraindication to rifampicin, Ceftriaxone can be prescribed:

- < 12yo: 125mg IM once only.
- > 12yo: 250 mg IM once only.
- Reconstitute 1g vial with 3.2ml lignocaine 1% (250 mg/ml).

OR

Ciprofloxacin, if the person is over 12 years old – 500 mg, oral, as a single dose.

For more information, see:

http://www.rch.org.au/clinicalguide/guideline_index/Meningococcal_Prophylaxis/

For your notes and thoughts

Safe prescribing station: case 8

Otitis media

Information given to the candidate

Peter has been brought to the surgery by his mother. He has been crying at night and unsettled during the day for the past week. You have diagnosed bilateral otitis media.

Name: Peter Gold

DOB: 16/09/2011

Address: 29 Park Avenue, Worthing BN11 2DH

Hospital/NHS No: ABc1234

Weight: 11 kg

Your task

You need to write a prescription in four minutes and then discuss your prescription and choice of treatment with the examiner for two minutes.

You have six minutes to complete the station; a warning bell will be given at five minutes.

Using the sample FP10 on p106, please write the prescription as in the examination.

Questions

What is your working diagnosis and why have you chosen this prescription?

What are the side effects?

Safe prescribing points?

What instructions or advice would you give Peter's parents?

What is expected from the candidate

The candidate should:
- introduce themself to the examiner
- provide fluent and structured answers
- write a clear and legible prescription
- choose an appropriate drug
- state the correct dose and the correct route of administration for the correct duration
- follow a systematic approach to get information from the BNFC
- demonstrate a knowledge of comorbidities, side effects, indications and contraindications
- explain in clear and simple language.

Answers

What is your working diagnosis and why have you chosen this prescription?
- Otitis media – Peter has been unwell for a week and is not improving.
- **Prescription:** Amoxicillin suspension.

What are the side effects?
- Nausea, vomiting, diarrhoea.
- Contraindication: penicillin hypersensitivity.

Safe prescribing points?
- Check for penicillin allergy – if Peter has never had it before, monitor him closely after the first dose for signs of allergy such as rash or wheezing. Ensure a treatment course length is prescribed.

What instructions or advice would you give Peter's parents?
- Give the complete course of medication.
- Use paracetamol as required if in pain or febrile.
- Drink plenty of fluids, and don't be too worried if Peter is off his food.
- Review with GP in four or five days if not recovered.

Copy of 'correct' prescription.

Pharmacy Stamp	Age	Title, Forename, Surname & Address
	1 yr 6 month.	Mr Peter Gold
	D.o.B	29 Park Av.
	16.09.2011	Worthing
Please don't stamp over age box	Wt. 11 kg	BN11 2DH
Number of days' treatment N.B. Ensure dose is stated	5	NHS Number: ABC 1234
Endorsements		

i. Amoxcillin oral suspension
125 mg/5 ml. Sugar free

125 mg three times a day. 5/7.

Supply 100 ml.

Signature of Prescriber	Date
A K Silver	03.03.2013

For dispenser No. of Prescns. on form

Dr A.K. Silver.
Worthing Practice
Worthing. BN11 4AB

Further information

Most ear infections occur in infants aged between six and 18 months, although anyone can get an ear infection. It is more common in boys than girls.

Symptoms and signs:

- Irritability.
- Poor feeding.
- Restlessness at night.
- Coughing.
- Runny nose.
- High temperature.
- Unresponsiveness to quiet sounds.
- Loss of balance.

Most cases of otitis media are bacterial or viral.

Most infections clear up within a couple of days. Paracetamol or ibuprofen (appropriate for the child's age) can be used to relieve pain and high temperature.

Antibiotics are usually only required if symptoms persist or are particularly severe.

For more information, see:

http://www.nhs.uk/conditions/Otitis-media/Pages/Introduction.aspx

For your notes and thoughts

Safe prescribing station: case 9

Impetigo

Information given to the candidate

Kevin James brings his eight-month-old son, LeBron, to the surgery. Kevin reports that LeBron has developed crusting lesions around his nose and mouth over the past 48 hours. Kevin is concerned because the lesions have become golden and weepy. LeBron is otherwise well and has no past medical history. Kevin also has a three-year-old daughter and she is well. You diagnose impetigo.

Name: LeBron James

DOB: 05/12/2012

Address: 56 Cleveland Close, Oxford, OX3 1WW

Hospital/NHS No: C23456A

Weight: 8 kg

Your task

You need to write a prescription in four minutes and then discuss your prescription and choice of treatment with the examiner for two minutes.

You have six minutes to complete the station; a warning bell will be given at five minutes.

Using the sample FP10 on p106, please write the prescription as in the examination.

Questions

What is your working diagnosis and why have you chosen this prescription?

What are the side effects?

What instructions or advice would you give LeBron's parents?

What is expected from the candidate

The candidate should:

- introduce themself to the examiner
- provide fluent and structured answers
- write a clear and legible prescription
- choose an appropriate drug
- state the correct dose and the correct route of administration for the correct duration
- follow a systematic approach to get information from the BNFC
- demonstrate a knowledge of comorbidities, side effects, indications and contraindications
- explain in clear and simple language.

Answers

What is your working diagnosis and why have you chosen this prescription?

- Impetigo.
- **Prescription:** Local/topical application of fucidic acid, 2% – good activity against staphalococci.

What are the side effects?

- Occasionally fucidic acid can cause hypersensitivity reactions.
- Avoid eyes as it can cause irritation.

What instructions or advice would you give LeBron's parents?

- LeBron should be kept away from nursery or play group.
- His sister should be monitored for similar lesions.
- Hands should be washed before and after applying medication.

Copy of 'correct' prescription.

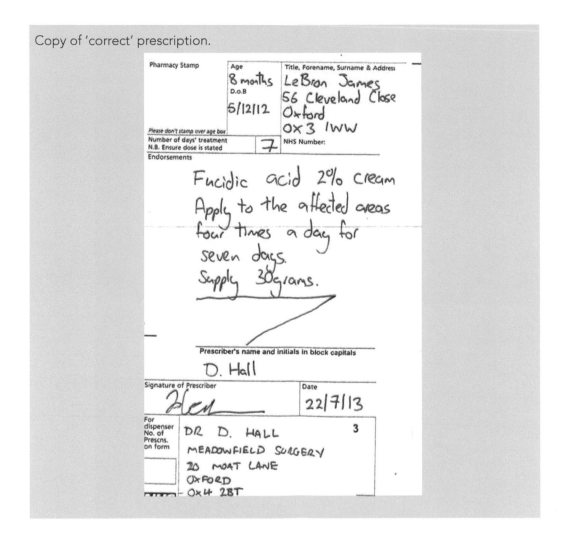

Further information

Impetigo is caused by Staphylococcus aureus and can be treated with a short course of topical fusidic acid.

Advice: The infection will resolve spontaneously within two to three weeks but treatment is appropriate if there is a danger of the infection being transmitted eg. to siblings.

Oral antibiotics such as flucloxacillin should be used if the infection is extensive, longstanding or child systemically unwell.

The child's finger nails should be kept short and they should be encouraged not to scratch the infected areas of skin.

The parents should wash their hands before and after applying the topical preparations to the infected area. Sharing towels should also be discouraged.

Any siblings should be monitored for similar signs of infection.

Parents should be advised that the child should be kept away from school or nursery whilst they are being treated for impetigo.

Cautions: Avoid contact with eyes, wash hands before and after applying to the child's skin.

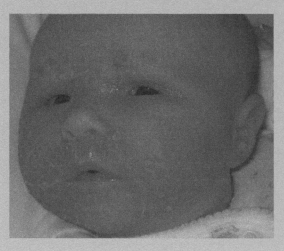

For your notes and thoughts

Safe prescribing station: case 10

Diarrhoea and vomiting

Information given to the candidate

Alice Martins has come to your practice with her 18-month-old daughter, Megan. Megan has been passing greenish, watery stools frequently for the past 36 hours and has vomited once. Megan appears miserable and tired. She is still having wet nappies, although her mother noticed that the frequency is reduced.

Name: Megan Martin

DOB: 14/02/2012

Address: The Mews, Grantham Avenue, Sheffield, SN4 7TF

Hospital/NHS No: A45678B

Weight: 9 kg

Your task

You need to write a prescription in four minutes and then discuss your prescription and choice of treatment with the examiner for two minutes.

You have six minutes to complete the station; a warning bell will be given at five minutes.

Using the FP10 sample on p106, please write the prescription as in the examination.

Questions

What is your working diagnosis and why have you chosen this prescription?

What are the side effects?

What instructions or advice would you give Megan's parents?

What is expected from the candidate

The candidate should:

- introduce themself to the examiner
- provide fluent and structured answers
- write a clear and legible prescription
- choose an appropriate drug
- state the correct dose and the correct route of administration for the correct duration
- follow a systematic approach to get information from the BNFC
- demonstrate a knowledge of comorbidities, side effects, indications and contraindications
- explain in clear and simple language.

Answers

What is your working diagnosis and why have you chosen this prescription?

- Gastroenteritis.
- **Prescription:** Oral rehydration solution – Megan is not vomiting and her dehydration is mild, as evidenced by decreased wet nappies.

What are the side effects?

- None.
- The child may be reluctant to drink the solution due to its taste.

What instructions or advice would you give Megan's parents?

- Reassure them that gastroenteritis is self-limiting.
- Reconstitute solution as instructed.
- Give her frequent, small drinks.

Copy of 'correct' prescription.

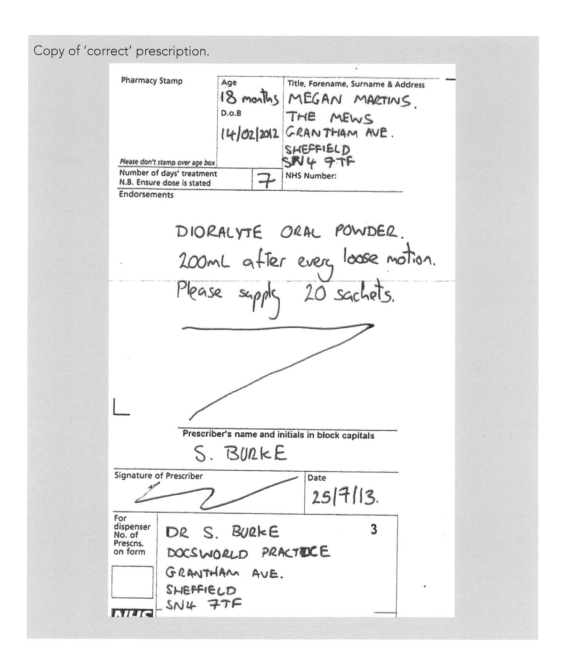

Further information

Reassure the parents that diarrhoea is usually self-limiting and will stop in due course.

For administration of oral rehydration therapy, reconstitute one sachet with 200ml of water, which should be freshly boiled and cooled for infants.

Alternatively, five sachets can be reconstituted in one litre of water. After reconstitution, the unused solution can be kept in the fridge for up to 24 hours and then discarded.

For your notes and thoughts